Working in a Medical Office Environment

Ann Vadala

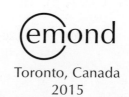

emond

Toronto, Canada
2015

Emond Montgomery Publications Limited
60 Shaftesbury Avenue
Toronto ON M4T 1A3
http://www.emp.ca

Printed in Canada.

We acknowledge the financial support of the Government of Canada through the Canada Book Fund for our publishing activities.

Emond Montgomery Publications has no responsibility for the persistence or accuracy of URLs for external or third-party Internet websites referred to in this publication, and does not guarantee that any content on such websites is, or will remain, accurate or appropriate.

Contributing writer: Melinda Vanzanten
Publisher: Mike Thompson
Managing editor, development: Kelly Dickson
Director, editorial and production: Jim Lyons
Developmental editor: Rachelle Redford
Copy and production editor: Francine Geraci
Production editor: Laura Bast
Permissions editor: Monika Schurmann
Proofreader: Rohini Herbert
Indexer: Paula Pike
Text designer: Shani Sohn
Cover designer: Tara Wells
Cover image: © Tetra Images / Alamy

Library and Archives Canada Cataloguing in Publication

Vadala, Ann, author
    Working in a medical office environment / Ann Vadala.

Includes index.
ISBN 978-1-55239-559-2 (pbk.)

    1. Medical offices—Canada—Management.   2. Medical assistants—Canada.
3. Medical secretaries—Canada.   I. Title.

R728.8.V33 2015   651'.961   C2014-905334-7

Contents

3 The Medical Office Environment

4 Medical Records 1: Legal Framework and Requirements

5 Medical Records 2: Chart Components, Organization, and Filing Systems

6 Scheduling

7 Diagnostics, Medical Imaging, and Common Medical Tests

8 Medical Office Pharmacology

Preface

An aging population and new medical advances have created exciting opportunities for medical professionals in both medical office and hospital care settings. Those who choose the fast-paced and fulfilling career path of health care administration in Canada are expected to have a broad scope of medical knowledge and a clear understanding of how to run a medical office. From patient management to billing, and everything in between, working in this profession is never dull.

Working in a Medical Office Environment is designed to provide detailed and practical information on how to run a medical office as a medical office administrator. The focus is on efficiency, effectiveness, and self-care tactics, in addition to core medical knowledge for superior patient care in what can be a hectic and stressful environment. Numerous features, like Did You Know boxes, scenarios, and practice tips, provide more in-depth background knowledge and context.

A variety of review questions—True or False, Fill in the Blank, Multiple Choice, and Short Answer—solidify new knowledge. Hybrid Learning activities are designed to access online learning resources and connect with other students for a teamwork learning experience that supports the skills necessary for a career in the medical office. End-of-chapter Activities are in-depth, practical skill–based questions, and require some research and collaboration.

The text is divided into ten chapters, with each chapter building on the information in the previous one. The learning outcomes at the start of each chapter clearly outline what students can expect to have learned by the completion of that chapter.

Chapter 1 is a key introductory chapter that outlines various positions within a medical office and the roles and duties of each. Education, training, skills, and abilities required for these positions are covered in detail, as are self-care strategies, such as how to effectively deal with stress and workplace safety issues.

Chapter 2 departs from the practical focus of the rest of the text by providing the history of health care in Canada and an overview of the current health care system. The chapter outlines the roles of the various levels of medical care and the acts of Parliament that constitute the country's health care responsibilities to its citizens.

Chapter 3 focuses on office structure and function. It reviews the legal aspects of the office environment, such as workplace health and safety regulations, as well as office security of both medical equipment and personnel. Office setup and ergonomics and their impact on employee efficiency and safety are also outlined. The specifics of maintaining a proper inventory for a medical office and creating a policy and procedure manual are also covered.

Chapters 4 and 5 provide detailed information on medical records—legal documents that are protected by two government privacy acts and that may also be required in legal proceedings. Chapter 4 deals with the legal and privacy aspects of medical documentation, while Chapter 5 is a practical, step-by-step guide of how to create, maintain, administer, and finally dispose of medical charts with an eye to legal and efficient filing and retrieval.

Chapter 6 is devoted to the complex and myriad systems of patient scheduling. The chapter opens with an explanation of the various scheduling types, with pros and cons, and then offers practical advice with supporting scenarios and practice tips for scheduling based on patient needs and medical urgency. The chapter also offers suggestions for how to deal with challenging patients while still maintaining efficiency and professionalism.

Diagnostic testing is the cornerstone of Chapter 7. Students are coached on how to fill in medical testing requisitions with information on the role of diagnostic testing in patient care. The chapter rounds out the subject with details on patient preparation, as well as test results procedures.

Although a large part of a medical office administrator's role is administration—that is, the efficient running of an office environment—the importance of a firm understanding of medicine can't be overstated. Chapter 8 is devoted to providing a thorough foundation in medical pharmacology. The legal aspects of drugs, terminology, classifications, forms, prescriptions, and storage and disposal best practices are all covered in depth in this chapter.

Medical billing is an essential part of any successful medical office and the intricacies of billing as a health care claim in Canada are discussed in detail in Chapter 9. The complexity of medical billing in Canada can be overwhelming; however, this chapter offers students a straightforward approach, with many opportunities to practise their learning.

Although the bulk of *Working in a Medical Office Environment* is devoted to medical office procedures, one important role of medical office administrators is working in a hospital setting as a unit clerk. In this role, being able to transcribe medical orders efficiently and with a very high degree of accuracy is critical. After completing Chapter 10, students will understand the role of a unit clerk, how to create and maintain hospital charts, medical symbols, and abbreviations, and how to correctly transcribe medical orders. This book is designed to give students the foundational knowledge necessary to launch them into a career in medical office administration.

Acknowledgments

Special thanks to the reviewers for their valuable comments and suggestions:

Lynn Berry, Algonquin College
Wendy Fisher, Mohawk College
Frances Jeffery, Durham College
Debbie Gamracy, Fanshawe College
Lisa Walters, Nova Scotia Community College

Inside the Medical Office: Roles, Responsibilities, and Skills

1

LEARNING OUTCOMES

After completing this chapter, you should be able to:

- describe the roles, duties, and responsibilities of medical office administrators (MAs)
- briefly describe the roles of other administrative health care staff in a medical office
- identify practical skills, soft skills, and interpersonal skills for MAs
- identify and apply time management skills
- define stress and identify strategies to reduce stress
- explain how MAs can keep current regarding medical knowledge, policies, and procedures, and the latest trends in the medical community

You can teach a student a lesson for a day; but if you can teach him to learn by creating curiosity, he will continue the learning process as long as he lives.

— Clay P. Bedford

Introduction

A competent and professional medical office administrator (MA) is essential for the efficient management of a medical office and is among a physician's greatest assets. A typical day might include advancing an appointment to allow an anxious parent to bring in a sick child, calming a patient who is angry about a bill, building a rapport with a patient who is afraid of being in a medical environment, or offering a listening ear to a patient—especially one who is elderly or lives alone and may be longing for contact. Every day is different and exciting and offers challenges. A career as a medical office administrator is a demanding one that requires dedication, commitment, and a strong desire to become a caregiver.

Medical office administration requires skills and expertise in patient greeting and registration; health card validation; telephone communication; scheduling; records management; billing, payroll, and financial management; **referrals**; insurance forms; and a range of correspondence. Other tasks may include preparing the patient and the examination room and possibly assisting the physician during the patient's office visit; sterilizing equipment and the waiting room (especially the children's area and toys); controlling inventory and ordering supplies; collecting and preparing laboratory specimens; and organizing meetings, conferences, and business trips.

This book introduces you to the role of the medical office administrator (also called a medical office assistant) within the broader health care system. In this chapter, we will look at the roles of various individuals who work together in a medical office to ensure its smooth functioning. We will then look at the role of the medical office administrator in more detail, including the initial and ongoing training and education required, areas of responsibility, and the specific skills you will need in order to succeed in this career.

Roles Within the Medical Office

In addition to the physician(s), a typical medical office includes a medical office manager, a medical office administrator/assistant, a receptionist, and a billing clerk. Depending on the office, some of these roles may be shared; for example, the office administrator may also perform the duties of a receptionist.

Table 1.1 sets out sample job descriptions for some of the above roles. Figure 1.1 shows a sample hierarchy of a typical medical office.

Medical Office Manager

The medical office manager is responsible for ensuring that the office runs smoothly and efficiently on a day-to-day basis. To this end, he or she oversees and implements organizational and clerical tasks and procedures, providing for uniformity in patient care and office procedures, such as appointment booking, maintaining a calendar, meeting support, administering and monitoring billing, and accounts receivable and payable. The manager is also responsible for ordering, maintaining, and tracking office and medical supplies.

TABLE 1.1   Medical Office Job Descriptions

Medical Office Manager	Medical Office Administrator	Medical Office Receptionist
Oversees financial matters, including payroll, bookkeeping, assisting the doctor(s) in developing and maintaining a budget, and banking	Acts as the liaison between the patient and the practitioner; provides all patient communication	Comforts patients by anticipating their anxieties, answering questions, and maintaining the reception area
Acts as the main point of contact for staff in matters of pay, benefits, and hours worked and makes decisions in accordance with policies established by the doctors	Maintains electronic medical records (EMRs)—updates addresses, allergies, phone numbers, etc., on each visit; ensures patients' records are up to date and correct regarding medications, treatments, symptoms, side effects, etc.	Keeps patient appointments on schedule
Develops and implements organizational policies and procedures for the facility or medical unit	Ensures that correct billing information is collected to produce and generate clean claims for submission; processes billing	Answers questions or provides general information, or may direct a patient to a person who can provide the information
Recommends, plans, and implements pay structure revisions	Schedules patient appointments	Schedules equipment service and repairs
Develops, recommends approval of, and maintains staff hours and vacation schedules	Schedules patients for tests and follow-up appointments promptly and efficiently	Ensures availability of treatment information by filing and retrieving patient records
Provides advice to the doctor(s) on finance, human resources, and other administrative matters	Prepares examination rooms; selects, sets up, and maintains medical supplies and equipment for all examinations and procedures	Greets patients when they enter the clinic
Ensures that staff are kept informed of current legislation, standards of practice, and scope of practice	Maintains business office inventory and supply inventory for exam rooms	Optimizes patients' satisfaction, provider time, and treatment room utilization by scheduling appointments in person or by telephone
Directs, supervises, and evaluates work activities of staff	Maintains patient privacy and confidentiality at all times	Answers telephones; responds to and sends faxes
Establishes work schedules and assignments for staff	Provides administrative support to practitioner, including reception, data entry, records maintenance, and correspondence	Protects patients' rights by maintaining confidentiality of personal and financial information
Maintains awareness of advances in medicine, computerized diagnostic and treatment equipment, data processing technology, government regulations, health insurance changes, and financing options	Coordinates flow of patient care; ensures that patient moves from waiting room to exam room and other clinic services without unnecessary delay	Processes incoming and outgoing mail (including email and faxes)

Managers have the responsibility of keeping health care as consistent as possible to ensure the best outcome for all patients. Because each patient and each complaint or concern may be slightly different, some flexibility must be given to the managers to adapt office protocol and procedures to patient needs. For example, if a patient regularly comes in for a blood pressure (BP) check on Wednesday mornings (current scheduling protocol for such quick

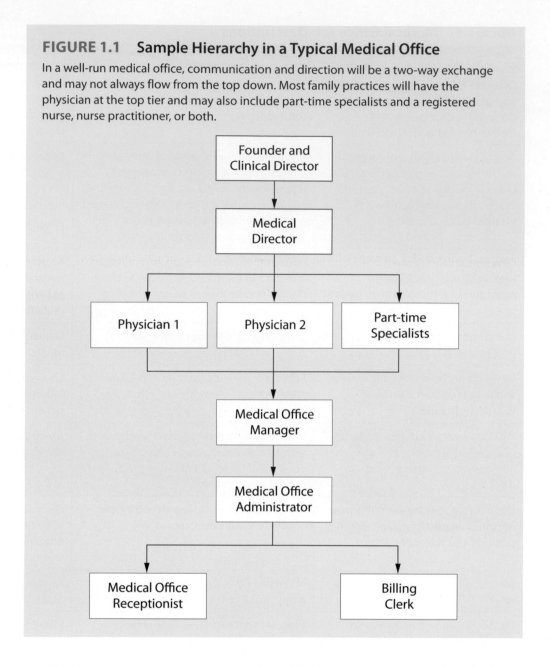

FIGURE 1.1   Sample Hierarchy in a Typical Medical Office

In a well-run medical office, communication and direction will be a two-way exchange and may not always flow from the top down. Most family practices will have the physician at the top tier and may also include part-time specialists and a registered nurse, nurse practitioner, or both.

checks) but is feeling dizzy on Friday and would like to come in then, office scheduling protocol needs to be flexible enough to accommodate this patient.

A medical office manager holds, at minimum, a medical office administration diploma combined with several years' experience as a medical office administrator/assistant and, often, further education. If you thrive on solving problems, supervising many different people, and organizing and streamlining processes, you might consider a career in medical office management after gaining experience as a medical office administrator.

Medical Office Administrator/Medical Office Assistant

The medical office administrator (MA), also called a medical office assistant, administrative medical assistant, or medical secretary, is the main link between the medical office and the public. Medical office administrators' responsibilities are largely clerical in nature, and training includes developing expertise in the following areas:

- records management
- procedure and diagnosis coding
- telephone procedures
- scheduling
- mail processing
- the completion and submission of medical billing and insurance forms
- all types of correspondence, including transcribing dictations
- chart management

MAs may work in a variety of health care settings, including physicians' offices, walk-in clinics, community health units, and hospitals; nursing homes; medical supply companies; chiropractic, podiatry, and physiotherapy clinics; medical insurance offices; veterinary hospitals; and universities. In some offices, performance of some routine clinical tasks may also be required.

A medical office administrator or assistant holds a medical office administration diploma and, usually, minimal experience (one to two years). We will examine the role of the MA in more detail in the rest of this chapter.

DID YOU KNOW?

In a hospital setting, a medical office administrator may take on the role of unit clerk (also known as a ward clerk) (see Chapter 10). Unit clerks play a vital role on hospital nursing units by performing such functions as transcribing physicians' orders, serving as a first point of contact for patients' families, scheduling patients for tests and treatments, and maintaining medical records for inpatients.

Medical Office Receptionist

A receptionist's major role in the medical office is greeting patients and other visitors. The patients' first contact with the office may be by phone or in person, and it will be the receptionist's job to obtain the information needed to begin a new chart or book an appointment. Once the patient or visitor has arrived at the office, the receptionist is responsible for putting the visitor at ease, obtaining his or her medical insurance information (e.g., OHIP), and directing him or her to the waiting area. Receptionists may also play a role in records management, referrals, and outgoing calls.

A receptionist may have a two-year medical office administration diploma or a one-year general office administration certificate. Some medical offices will accept a high-school diploma, but remuneration will reflect education level.

Although the role of receptionist is typically a separate role in a medical office, some offices—particularly smaller practices—may not have a receptionist on staff, and receptionist duties may fall to the MA.

Billing Clerk

The billing clerk focuses on diagnostic and procedure coding and billing. Billing clerks complete insurance claim forms and determine insurance coverage and limitations for patients.

A billing clerk holds a medical office administration diploma. Generally, billing responsibilities fall to the MA in addition to his or her other tasks. However, in large offices, an MA may work solely as a billing clerk.

BOX 1.1	The Medical Office Administrator

A medical office administrator (MA) or receptionist is the front line of the medical office. Individuals in these roles are an important link in Canadian health care, serving as the first point of contact for patients and visitors to the office, clinic, floor, or other workplace setting, and contributing to its overall operation.

An important part of your job as an MA involves carrying out your duties in accordance with the range of legal and ethical responsibilities that physicians have under federal and provincial/territorial legislation and the regulations developed by various governing bodies, such as the College of Physicians and Surgeons of Ontario. If, in dealing with medical records, you fail to protect the confidentiality of patients' personal information, for example, the physician will be in breach of his or her legal obligations under the *Personal Health Information Protection Act*, and serious consequences may follow.

One important limit on your responsibilities flows from the fact that in Canada, only licensed physicians are permitted by law to give medical advice to patients. This means that if administrative staff offer medical or medication advice, both the physician and the MA may find themselves involved in a medical malpractice lawsuit. The MA may, however, ensure that the patient understands directions given by the physician in regard to medications, treatment, or tests. We will examine legal responsibilities in more detail in other chapters of this text.

Typical work hours for MAs are 37.5 to 40 hours per week, with some working part time. Unlike many general office administrators, it is rare for MAs to work from home because their presence is essential to the smooth running of the medical setting.

Table 1.2 summarizes the primary administrative and clinical responsibilities of MAs.

DID YOU KNOW?

The first MAs were most likely the physician's spouse or neighbour, who fell into the position of helping the physician meet the needs of both the patients and the office. Today's MAs are skilled and versatile professionals who play an integral role in a medical office, working closely with the physicians, nursing staff, other medical staff, and patients.

Education and Training

Educational requirements vary by employer. However, most employers prefer at least a two-year college office administration diploma with a medical concentration. Specific types of medical office administration may require supplementary training or education. For example, a unit/ward clerk will also be given in-hospital training before managing a hospital floor's nursing station or nursing centre, while an MA working in a specialist's office may require upgrading in medical terminology specific to that specialty.

The Ontario Ministry of Training, Colleges and Universities publishes program standards for every Medical Office Administration program.[1] These standards bring a greater degree of consistency to medical office administration programs Ontario-wide. Other provinces have their own ministry guidelines for colleges, universities, and training centres.

Ongoing professional development will help you acquire the additional skills you may need depending on your career path, and will ensure that your professional knowledge remains up to date. Additional training may be obtained from various sources. The Ontario Hospital Association provides professional development for medical office administrators, as does the Association of Administrative Assistants. The Institute for Healthcare Improvement is American but an excellent online resource.

TABLE 1.2   Primary Administrative and Clinical Responsibilities of MAs

Administrative Responsibilities	Clinical Responsibilities
Answering telephones	Helping the patient prepare for examinations and other procedures*
Scheduling appointments	Recording medical history
Interviewing and instructing new patients	Assisting in examinations when requested to do so*
Coding and transmitting insurance claims	Cleaning and sterilizing instruments and equipment*
Explaining fees	Instructing patients regarding preparation for radiologic and laboratory examinations*
Opening and sorting mail	Keeping supply cabinets and examining rooms well stocked*
Answering routine correspondence	Performing a variety of laboratory tests, such as urinalysis* and blood studies
Transcribing electronic dictation	
Coding and transmitting insurance	
Maintaining financial records and files	
Supervising personnel	
Helping with the preparation of speeches	
Clipping articles from professional journals	
Conducting journal article research	

* Clinical skills usually required of the office assistant/administrator

Skills and Abilities of the Medical Office Administrator

Being responsible for the day-to-day administration of any medical setting requires knowledge, commitment, and patience; a high level of professionalism; and practical skills as well as soft skills. As an MA, you will interact with people and will need specific skills to perform the full range of activities that will be required of you. Mastering these will prepare you to offer excellent customer service and maintain a pleasant office environment for both your co-workers and your clients.

Practical Skills

Practical skills include general, administrative, and clinical skills, such as keyboarding and filing.

MAs must have up-to-date computer skills and must be able to use word-processing software (such as Microsoft Word), spreadsheets (such as Microsoft Excel), and databases (such as Microsoft Access). They must be able to troubleshoot basic computer malfunctions and be able to obtain valid information from reliable online sources. Knowledge of medical terminology and basic pharmacology is necessary for the MA to be able to communicate with physicians, patients, and pharmacy staff. As mentioned, knowledge of medico-legal matters (those relating to law as well as medicine) is also vital to avoiding medical liability suits.

Table 1.3 lists the practical skills that MAs must possess to run an office efficiently.

TABLE 1.3   Practical Skills of MAs

General Skills	Administrative Skills	Clinical Skills
Medical terminology, usage, and spelling	Telephone skills and scheduling	Application of aseptic technique and infection control*
Basics of medical law and ethics	Proficiency in typing and keyboarding	Testing for vital signs
Human relations and personal communications	Communication, both written and spoken	Interviewing and recording of patient history
Computer literacy	Electronic dictation and word processing	Patient instruction*
Documentation of health information	Health information and management	Specimen collection and handling*
Cardiopulmonary resuscitation	Patient and insurance billing	Performance of selected tests
Legible handwriting		
Emergency first aid kit		

* Clinical skills usually required of the office assistant/administrator

Soft Skills

In addition to the practical skills listed above, a successful MA will require a range of **soft skills**. These are skills that employers and patients value, and that allow MAs to work effectively when working alone and positively when working with others. Following is a list of soft skills that will serve you well in your career.

- *Motivation, Initiative, and Responsibility*
  An MA who takes initiative demonstrates to the physician that he or she is motivated and satisfied with the job. Office staff should be willing to help others, if able, and willing to learn additional skills. For example, perhaps the receptionist has a line-up of patients, some needing to check in and others needing to rebook an appointment. As an MA, you might volunteer to take over the patients checking in so that the receptionist can focus on rebooking appointments. Or, perhaps you notice that the physician has left a pile of charts on the desk that are no longer needed. Without having to be asked, you might take initiative by quietly removing and filing them.

  A responsible office employee arrives on time and is available for all scheduled worked hours.

- *Attitude, Empathy, and Listening*
  A positive attitude plays an important role in wellness—not only yours, but patients' too. You should be able to accept constructive criticism that is provided to help you excel professionally.

  Being able to put yourself in your patients' situations and see their point of view will help you understand how they feel and may offer insight into why they may be angry or upset. This understanding allows you to look at situations objectively and not be personally offended.

SCENARIO 1.1

Your morning has been very busy with lots of interruptions, and you are feeling frazzled. A patient approaches the desk and angrily states, "I have been waiting a long time to be seen. How much longer? Patients who arrived after me have come and gone!" You realize that in all the confusion, you did not place this patient's chart into the proper pile, and the physician believes that she was a "no show." What do you do? How will you defuse the patient's anger? What will you say to the physician?

SCENARIO 1.2

Your physician went overtime with the first patient of the day and has been unable to make up the time during the morning appointments. Now it is time for the office to close for lunch, and there are two patients yet to be seen in the waiting room. Both patients have been waiting over 30 minutes for their scheduled appointments. One of the patients approaches you. He is angry at the long wait and demands an explanation, plus an idea of how much longer the wait will be. The patient is frustrated, and his tone and body language are aggressive. Put yourself in the patient's place. How would you respond? Would you be able to defuse some of the patient's anger? Is there anything you might do to make the patient's wait more comfortable?

Patients expect receptionists and assistants to have the answers and be able to help solve their problems. Thus, they may view staff who cannot provide answers as antagonistic or indifferent. Listen and observe. Learn to evaluate patients' behaviour. Listen to what they are saying, both verbally and with their body language. Use these clues to decide on the best response.

- *Cultural Awareness and Sensitivity*
  An awareness of and sensitivity to cultural diversity is an extremely important soft skill to develop. Patients' value systems, beliefs, and practices—like your own—are influenced by, among other things, their nationality, ethnic origin, gender, age, religion, sexual orientation, disability, and socio-economic status. Language barriers may create obvious difficulties with communication, while other differences may affect your interactions in more subtle ways. It is important to be aware of how this may affect communication and to treat all patients with equal respect.

- *Communication*
  Communicating effectively with patients is important to providing high-quality care. Do not dismiss the importance of non-verbal communication. Be aware of the patient's body language and facial expressions for clues as to how relaxed or stressed he or she may be. Listen to the patient's concerns and speak clearly. Also, be aware of your own body language and the effect it may have on patients as well as your co-workers.

- *Appearance*
  The essentials of a professional appearance are good health, good grooming, good posture, and appropriate dress. A well-groomed MA in appropriate workplace attire has a positive psychological effect on patients and contributes to the perception of professional competence.

- *Confidentiality*
  The ability to keep information confidential not only instills trust but also is essential for ensuring that you meet the legal requirements placed on those who handle patients' personal information.

PRACTICE TIP

Increasing your awareness and understanding of diversity will result in improved communication and interactions with patients.

- *Critical Thinking Skills*

  The best employees apply **critical thinking skills**. Critical thinkers are aware of alternatives to solving problems and can think "outside the box." They are resourceful and are able to break down problems or questions into smaller parts, and then examine these parts to find solutions or reach alternative conclusions about a problem or an issue. Critical thinkers use good judgment to solve problems based on knowledge and experience.

SCENARIO 1.3

Suppose you feel that your medical office should have an additional phone line, as there are periods during the day when the lines are busy and you are unable to call out. This hampers your ability to call patients regarding follow-up and to keep up with referral requests. You have spoken to the physician, and she is not willing to pay for a new line. How would you solve your dilemma?

- *Teamwork*

  The ability to work in a team is essential to the smooth operation of a medical office. Tasks are coordinated to flow from one to the other, and the office staff must work together to ensure patients' charts are up to date, patients' needs are met, and wait times are minimized. It is important to remember that team dynamics often change. Changes may occur when a new employee is hired or a physician retires, for example. The ability to adapt to these changes requires flexibility and a willingness to adapt.

- *Time Management*

  Developing excellent time management skills will allow you to complete multiple tasks in an efficient manner. MAs should be able to prioritize and perform multiple tasks, allowing the physician to focus on spending more time with patients.

BOX 1.2   Time Management Strategies

Here are some specific strategies that will help you increase your efficiency and improve your time management skills.

- *Set goals and deadlines for work to be completed.* Stay motivated by measuring your progress and offering yourself an incentive for each goal or deadline reached. Manage large and complicated projects by breaking them down into smaller parts and then setting deadlines for completing each part.

- *Streamline all repetitive tasks.* Never do the same thing twice. Use templates, macros, and other shortcuts provided by computer software.

- *Handle time wasters.* Stay focused on the task at hand. Let co-workers know that you need uninterrupted time to complete your work. If you have an office, shut your door. Do not encourage chit-chat. It may take several tries to persuade co-workers that you have work to complete and do not want to be interrupted. Remove any items or obstacles that will make it difficult for you to focus. Avoid procrastination.

- *Make **downtime** productive.* Set time aside each day to complete routine tasks, such as filing. Organize files and emails; help out a co-worker who is swamped with work; read or upgrade your skills; engage in professional development through further training.

- *Neatness and Organization.* Neatness not only conveys an impression of professionalism but will help you stay organized and allow you to carry out tasks, such as accessing documents and meeting deadlines, more easily. Use organizational aids and supplies, such as planners, incoming and outgoing trays, and file folders. Manage your workload by controlling paper and email. Use the flags and folders provided by your email program. Mark or file incoming mail as Items for Immediate Attention, Items to Deal with Later, Items to Be Forwarded, and Items to Be Filed.

PRACTICE TIP

As an MA, you will always be multitasking. Using a steno pad is an effective way to organize your to-do list and stay on task. The steno pad is a legal document in the medical office, one that may be used as a legal resource in the event of litigation and which may be stored for several years. Each MA in the office should have his or her own steno pad with name, start date, and finish date clearly written on the cover.

Dealing Effectively with Stress

Stress has been defined as a subjective phenomenon that creates worry or anxiety; a non-specific response of the body to change; and emotional, physical, or mental pressure. Stress is not always negative—in some cases, it may be helpful when it motivates people to accomplish more. Chronic workplace stress, however, is a serious health threat that can have devastating effects.

Stress can be categorized as low, normal, and high. When stress is too low, staff are not motivated and tend to be less productive. When stress is too high, staff are unable to cope and often become ill.

Without a certain amount of stress in the workplace, many tasks would not be accomplished. The trick is to find a balance so that stress remains at a manageable level. Stresses that are not considered normal and that often increase overall stress levels are noise, staff shortages, lack of control, conflicting work demands, harassment, and bullying. These stresses often lead to illness and poor work performance.

BOX 1.3   Signs of Difficulty in Coping with Stress

A range of symptoms can indicate that a person is having difficulty coping with stress:

- *Physical symptoms* can include headaches, teeth grinding or a clenched jaw, chest pain, shortness of breath, a pounding heart, high blood pressure, muscle aches, indigestion, constipation or diarrhea, increased perspiration, fatigue, insomnia, and a higher frequency of illness.
- *Psycho-social symptoms* may include anxiety, irritability, sadness, anger, mood swings, hypersensitivity, depression, slowed thinking or racing thoughts, feelings of helplessness or hopelessness, and decreased motivation.
- *Cognitive symptoms* may include decreased attention, difficulty concentrating, forgetfulness, and reduced problem-solving abilities.
- *Behavioural symptoms* may include overeating or loss of appetite, impatience, procrastination, increased use of alcohol or drugs, increased smoking, withdrawal or isolation from others, neglect of responsibility, poor personal hygiene, and change in close family relationships.

SOURCE: Based on "Workplace Stress," the Canadian Centre for Occupational Health and Safety.

You can limit some of the factors that lead to above-normal levels of stress by doing the following:

- *Take your breaks.* Do not skip lunch or other breaks during the day.
- *Move.* Get up from the computer and move around. Stretch. It is recommended that you take a movement break of 30 seconds for every hour spent working at your desk.

- While working, use these techniques at your desk:
  - *Slow your breathing:* Take deep breaths, holding your breath on inhalation and then releasing slowly. Repeat several times.
  - *Practise muscle relaxation:* Pick a muscle and slowly tense it, then release. Repeat tensing and relaxing two or three times for each location you are able to tense.
- *Report health and safety hazards,* as well as harassment or bullying. Take control.
- *Try to position your workspace* (e.g., computer, telephone) in a way that minimizes noise and distractions.
- *Ask for help.* If you are drowning in paperwork or are behind in filing, ask for help from a co-worker or the medical office manager.
- *Laugh.* Laughter is truly one of the best medicines.
- *Reward yourself* for meeting a deadline or completing a difficult task.

Outside of the office, some stress relievers include the following:

- *Sleep.* Getting eight hours of sleep will help you start a new day.
- *Exercise!* During exercise, bodies release endorphins, which create a natural high. Exercise helps regulate sleep, reduce tension, decrease depression, and boost your immune system.

NOTE

1. Search "medical office administration" at the ministry's website: http://www.tcu.gov.on.ca/eng.

RESOURCES

Ontario Hospital Association:
http://www.oha.com

Association of Administrative Assistants:
http://www.aaa.ca/index_e.php

The Institute for Healthcare Improvement:
http://www.ihi.org

REVIEW QUESTIONS

True or False?

1. Every employee and patient has the same idea about what "good" service means.
2. Administrative responsibilities and administrative skills are one and the same.
3. The ability to work as part of a team is not an essential skill for the medical office worker.
4. Stress always has a negative impact on work performance.
5. Critical thinkers break down problems into manageable parts.

Fill in the Blank

1. Outside of the office, _____ and _____ are critical stress relievers.
2. The first _____ were most likely the physician's spouse or neighbour, who fell into the position of helping the physician meet the needs of both the patients and the office.
3. A medical _____ is chiefly responsible for keeping the medical office running smoothly and efficiently.
4. Being able to put yourself in your patients' situation or understanding their point of view helps you understand how they feel or why they may be angry. This skill is known as _____.
5. Being responsible for the day-to-day administration of any medical setting requires knowledge, commitment, and patience, a high level of professionalism, and _____ skills as well as _____ skills.

Multiple Choice

Choose the best answer.

1. Which of the responsibilities below is NOT an administrative responsibility?
   a. answering telephones
   b. cleaning and sterilizing medical instruments and equipment
   c. scheduling appointments
   d. opening and sorting mail

2. Time management involves all of the below except
   a. setting goals and deadlines
   b. limiting stress
   c. teamwork and appearance
   d. communication and productivity

3. A medical office administrator is a versatile professional whose duties include
   a. advising patients regarding health care
   b. health card validation
   c. prescribing medications
   d. painting the examination room

4. If you are drowning in paperwork, you should
   a. quit
   b. ask for help from a co-worker
   c. pretend you never received the paperwork
   d. pass the responsibility for the paperwork on to your co-worker

5. Which of the following is NOT considered a soft skill?
   a. teamwork skills
   b. computer skills
   c. interpersonal skills
   d. communication skills

Short Answer

1. How could a manual or an electronic planner or calendar help you stay organized?

2. Is all stress bad? How can stress be helpful?

3. Define stress. Name one thing that has caused stress in your life.

4. Name four forms of communication. Identify and explain your strongest communication method.

5. Time management is important for the efficient operation of a medical office. Describe the two time management practices that you feel are the most important. Explain.

6. You have 15 minutes of free time. How will you spend that time wisely?

7. Your day has become extremely busy. You have not taken any breaks and are starting to feel tired and negative. What can you do in this situation?

8. Critical thinking skills are essential in a busy medical office. Give an example of a situation in which you had to employ critical thinking.

9. You are working in a medical office as a receptionist and a patient has arrived to check in. She is clearly stressed and emotional and is becoming verbally abusive. How do you handle the situation?

HYBRID LEARNING

Using Blackboard's online discussion board, provide a 200- to 300-word response, in paragraph form, to the following questions.

1. Browse the Association of Administrative Assistants' website and respond to the following:

   a. How do you become a member?

   b. Briefly describe three benefits that would influence you, as an MA, to become a member.

2. Describe a situation in which you have experienced stress in the workplace and how you handled that stressor. List ways in which you could have improved your handling of that situation. Provide helpful advice on one fellow classmate's experience.

ACTIVITIES

1. Soft skills are difficult to define and measure. They include a positive attitude and the ability to interact and communicate productively, solve problems, and manage your time. The chart below lists 12 soft skills. Work with your group to define each one, and give a workplace example. Finally, using a scale of 1 to 10 (10 being your strongest skill and 1 your weakest skill), rate yourself on each soft skill. The first item is given as an example.

Rating	Skill	Definition	Example
3	Motivation	helps guide and maintain goals	taking a course to enhance current knowledge of office procedures
	Communication		
	Positive attitude		
	Strong work ethic		
	Teamwork skills		
	Interpersonal skills		
	Integrity		
	Flexibility and adaptability		
	Problem solving		
	Empathy		
	Initiative		
	Neatness and organization		

2. Using the Association of Administrative Assistants' website, provide a description of the association, including its mission statement and some of the upcoming calendar events.

3. You have just secured a full-time job in a fast-paced medical office. Your hours of work are Monday to Friday from 8:00 a.m. to 4:00 p.m. each day, with a half-hour unpaid lunch. You start to notice that other employees are showing up late, leaving early, and taking extended breaks. How do you handle this situation?

4. Organize the following list of tasks and duties in order of priority on the planner provided. Using your time management skills, group similar tasks together to save time, and designate an approximate amount of time for each task. If you run out of time, list any tasks that you feel can be put off until tomorrow.

   Note: It is Tuesday, and the workday is from 8:00 a.m. to 4:00 p.m., with a half-hour lunch from 12:00 to 12:30. Time slots are 15 minutes each.

   List of tasks and duties:
   - Enter Dr. Lee's OHIP billing
   - Clean Reception toy area
   - Create new files for patients G. Wong, T. Vanduzen, T. Perry
   - Clean kitchen area
   - Stock examining room cabinets
   - Call next day morning appointment patients to confirm appointments
   - File morning patient files
   - Organize waiting room chairs
   - Cover Reception for Jamie from 1:00 to 1:30
   - Fax prescriptions to pharmacy from morning appointments
   - Book referral appointments for Dr. Lee from the morning
   - Update office manual with new protocols from last staff meeting
   - Book nursing interviews for next Friday (3 in total)
   - Update Dr. Lee's PPT medical rounds lecture in three weeks
   - Enter Dr. Nagy's OHIP billing
   - Tackle the old pile of non-urgent documents
   - Create new files for "renovations" and "invoices"

Task	Time Allotted	Time
		8:00–8:15
		8:15–8:30
		8:30–8:45
		8:45–9:00
		9:00–9:15
		9:15–9:30
		9:30–9:45
		9:45–10:00
		10:00–10:15
		10:15–10:30
		10:30–10:45
		10:45–11:00
		11:00–11:15
		11:15–11:30
		11:30–11:45
		11:45–12:00
Lunch	30 min	12:00–12:15
		12:15–12:30
		12:30–12:45
		12:45–1:00
Cover Reception for Jamie	30 min	1:00–1:15
		1:15–1:30
		1:30–1:45
		1:45–2:00
		2:00–2:15
		2:15–2:30
		2:30–2:45
		2:45–3:00
		3:00–3:15
		3:15–3:30
		3:30–3:45
		3:45–4:00

Tasks for tomorrow:

Canada's Health Care System

2

LEARNING OUTCOMES

After completing this chapter, you should be able to:

- summarize the history of the Canadian health care system

- outline the organizational structure of the Canadian health care system and the division of responsibilities between the federal government and the provinces

- explain the criteria and conditions for funding established by the *Canada Health Act*

- understand provincial insurance plans and insured and uninsured services

- identify various health care settings

- distinguish among primary, secondary, and tertiary levels of health care

- understand the different family practice models and their corresponding compensation models

- explain the latest developments in Canada's health care system and identify some challenges

[O]*ur noble tradition that no sick person of any age, sex, race or religion whatsoever, shall ever suffer for need of medical care on account of poverty or any other cause … should be based on our willingness to give, and should be construed as an act of our charity. It should not be exploited: nor should it be assumed as a God-given right by way of its beneficiaries.*

—Dr. J.H. MacDermot, Osler lecture, 1939

Introduction

Government-funded health care for medically necessary services is one of the defining characteristics of our society; patients receive treatment based on their needs, not their ability to pay. **Medicare** reflects the value we as a society in Canada place on fairness and equity.

The history of medicare in Canada is long and complex and has been influenced by many factors, including politics, social change, medical knowledge and technology, and economics. In the future, medicare will continue to evolve to reflect developments in health care service delivery, the cost of new technology, population demographics, and many other factors.

This chapter provides an overview of the development of Canada's health care system and the current delivery model. It also examines some of the challenges our health care system faces now and will face in the future.

History of Health Care in Canada

Since Canada became a country in 1867, responsibility for health care has been shared between the federal and the provincial/territorial governments. At the time of Confederation, the *British North America Act* (BNA Act) determined the responsibilities of each level of government. With respect to health care, under section 91, the federal government was designated responsibility for quarantine, the establishment and maintenance of marine hospitals, and Aboriginal peoples. Under section 91, the provinces were responsible for hospitals, asylums, charities, and charitable institutions. These responsibilities have changed over the years and will continue to evolve in the future.

> **DID YOU KNOW?**
>
> Recognizing the need for a national medical body in their newly created country, in October 1867, three months after Confederation, 164 physicians created the Canadian Medical Association (CMA). Today, the CMA is a national organization with over 76,000 members. It provides leadership to Canadian physicians and advocates for access to high-quality health care for all.

Early Years

Following Confederation, the Department of Agriculture oversaw federal health responsibilities. During and after the First World War, a range of social welfare issues came to the fore—including war casualties, poverty, poor housing, industrial accident rates, and high maternal and infant mortality rates—and the Canadian Medical Association (CMA) began to advocate for the creation of a federal department of health.[1] Other driving factors were high mortality rates from communicable diseases, such as tuberculosis and the Spanish influenza epidemic of 1918–1919. In 1919, a bill was passed in the House of Commons to create a federal Department of Health, which would aim to ensure "the conservation of the health of the people."[2]

Today, our health care system is mostly government funded; the federal government subsidizes the provinces through income tax paid by Canadian taxpayers. According to section 3 of the **Canada Health Act** (CHA), which will be discussed in more detail later in this chapter, the primary objective of Canadian health care policy is "to protect, promote and restore the physical and mental well-being of residents of Canada and to facilitate reasonable access to health services without financial or other barriers."

Prior to the Second World War, health care in Canada for the general population was, for the most part, funded and delivered privately. Patients paid physicians for medical services as they were delivered, and many could not afford the cost of care. Municipalities provided subsidies to local hospitals, and charities and churches encouraged doctors to provide their services for free to patients who could not afford to pay.[3] In contrast, a few Western European countries had already introduced health insurance—Germany in 1883 and Britain in 1911 for low-income workers.

DID YOU KNOW?

Early Canadian physicians were not necessarily wealthy members of the community. Often, they were paid in produce, not cash. For example, a physician might have been paid two chickens for a house call to treat a child with a cold. Physicians also bartered their services. For example, a family physician might "trade" services with a dentist.

In the 1920s, as Canada's population grew and the need for care became a more prominent issue, the CMA held conferences on medical services, at which speakers shared their views on the proposal for state-funded health insurance. Some provinces, including British Columbia and Saskatchewan, began to examine the possibility of health insurance more seriously. The response to the idea in Canada was generally mixed, ranging from support from public health advocates, workers, and farmers, to opposition from many practitioners. Many doctors believed that government involvement in the doctor–patient relationship would threaten physicians' status as independent professionals and create a situation in which they were "subservient" to the state.[4]

The First Provincial Plans

The Great Depression, which began in 1929, played a key role in the development of Canada's social welfare system, including the first provincial health insurance plans. Combined with drought and crop failures, the worldwide crisis had a particularly devastating effect on the Canadian West. In 1932, Canada's first socialist party, the Co-operative Commonwealth Federation (CCF), emerged. The CCF, which would eventually become the New Democratic Party, believed that government should take responsibility for social and economic planning and implement social welfare policies to eliminate inequality. Among the first members of the CCF elected to Parliament was Tommy Douglas, who became Saskatchewan's premier in 1944 (see Box 2.1).[5] In 1947, Saskatchewan became the first province to introduce universal public hospital insurance. British Columbia and Alberta implemented plans in the following years.

BOX 2.1　**Tommy Douglas**

Tommy Douglas emigrated from Scotland with his family in 1919, settling in Winnipeg. He was ordained as a minister and moved to Saskatchewan, where he witnessed the devastation of the Great Depression during the 1930s—including the struggles of those unable to pay for medical care—firsthand. He believed that political change was necessary to end the suffering of the poor, and vowed to work for change:

> It was in those days I made up my mind that if ever I had the power I would, if it were humanly possible, see that the financial barrier between those who needed health services and those who gave health services was forever removed.[6]

Douglas was premier in 1947, when Saskatchewan became the first province to offer hospital insurance by implementing the Hospital Services Plan. He resigned before the province's full medical insurance plan was passed in 1961, but he had been instrumental in its creation. He has been called the "greatest Canadian" by many, as well as the father of Canadian medicare.

The CCF left an important legacy in Canada's values and social policies, many of which were implemented by subsequent governments. In addition to medicare, these include the Canada-wide old age pension plan and unemployment insurance.

SOURCE: Based on "Tommy Douglas," by L.D. Lovick, 2013, *The Canadian Encyclopedia*, Historica Foundation, http://www.thecanadianencyclopedia.com.

Emergence of a National System

In 1957, the federal government passed the *Hospital Insurance and Diagnostic Services Act*. Under the Act, the federal government would cover one-half of the costs for certain hospital and diagnostic services for all of the provinces and territories. This new cost-sharing structure represented a significant development in Canadian health care, and by 1961, all provinces and territories were offering publicly funded inpatient hospital and diagnostic services.

The next development came in 1962, when Saskatchewan again became a pioneer, introducing the *Medical Care Insurance Act*, a provincial medical (as opposed to just a hospital) insurance plan. Doctors in the province fiercely opposed the plan and a strike ensued; many left the province to practise elsewhere. Meanwhile, the federal government had formed a Royal Commission on Health Services to study the possibility of creating a national medical insurance plan. In 1964, Supreme Court Justice Emmett Hall tabled the commission's report, known as the Hall Report.[7] The Hall Report recommended a national health care program for the country. Responsibility for the system, which would cover all hospital and preventive services for all Canadians, would be shared by the federal and provincial governments.

Two years later, in 1966, the *Medical Care Act* introduced by Lester B. Pearson's Liberal government was passed in the House of Commons by a vote of 177 to 2. Canada's national medicare system was born. The Act provided for 50/50 cost sharing between the federal and provincial governments for medical service costs. To receive the federal contribution, the provinces agreed to insure hospital and physician services. Neither the *Medical Care Act* nor the *Hospital Insurance and Diagnostic Services Act* explicitly prevented the provinces from charging patients directly. However, because federal assistance was proportional to what the province spent, any extra charges imposed by the province would be deducted from the federal contribution. This discouraged the provinces from extra-billing patients or applying other charges.[8]

By 1972, all provinces as well as the Yukon territory had universal medical insurance plans with federal cost sharing. In 1977, the cost-sharing arrangement was replaced by a block-funding model under the *Federal–Provincial Fiscal Arrangements and Established Programs Financing Act*. Under the new model, the federal government provided a sum of money to a province for a specified purpose (e.g., health expenses), providing greater flexibility in terms of how the funding could be invested.[9] With federal funding now separate from provincial government health expenditures, there was no longer a disincentive to apply direct patient charges. Physicians started extra-billing patients, demanding they make a cash payment in addition to the fees that would be reimbursed through the provincial health plan—a clear violation of the spirit of medicare. Many hospitals did the same. For example, hospitals in Newfoundland, New Brunswick, Quebec, Ontario, Saskatchewan, Alberta, and British Columbia applied user charges, and most provinces authorized extra-billing.[10]

The *Canada Health Act* defines **extra-billing** as the billing for an insured health service rendered to an insured person by a medical practitioner or a dentist in an amount in addition to any amount paid or to be paid for that service by the health care insurance plan of a province (for example, OHIP in Ontario). For example, if a physician charged a patient any amount for an insured office visit, then extra-billing was incurred. The *Canada Health Act* defines a **user charge** as any charge for an insured health service other than extra-billing that is permitted by a provincial or territorial health care insurance plan and is not payable by the plan. An example of a user charge would be a facility fee, such as accommodations or meals provided to an inpatient who requires chronic care and is a permanent resident in a hospital or other institution, or liquid nitrogen treatment for removing warts on the hands. (It is interesting to note that liquid nitrogen treatment for warts on the feet or genitals is covered by OHIP.) Both services are billed directly to the patient.

Despite federal funding and universal access to care, differences existed among the provinces in terms of what, specifically, was covered by the insurance plans. In a Health Services Review report released in 1980, Justice Emmett Hall expressed concern over the extra-billing and user charges that some physicians and hospitals were applying. Hall found that equitable access to care was threatened by these practices, and the following year, a House of Commons Task Force on Federal–Provincial Fiscal Arrangements concluded that the federal funding arrangement was adequate and that these practices were detrimental to the system.

The Canada Health Act

In 1984, Canada passed the *Canada Health Act*, a relatively brief Act that combines the *Hospital Insurance and Diagnostic Services Act* and the *Medical Care Act*. Despite its name, the CHA applies to the provinces and territories. Specifically, it sets out five criteria (discussed below) that provinces and territories must meet to quality for the full Canada Health Transfer (CHT) paid by the federal government under the *Federal–Provincial Fiscal Arrangements and Established Programs Financing Act*. It also outlines the penalties that the federal health minister may apply to provinces that fail to meet the requirements of the CHA. The CHA does not regulate service delivery, and it does not ban or regulate the private purchasing of health care services.

Criteria for Federal Funding

To qualify for the full Canada Health Transfer cash contribution in a given year, a province or territory must satisfy the following criteria, set out in sections 8 through 12 of the Act:

1. **Public administration:** The insurance plan must be administered by a public authority (referred to as a "single payer") that operates on a not-for-profit basis and that is accountable to the provincial government. This criterion, unlike the following four, focuses on the administration of health services and not on the patient.
2. **Comprehensiveness:** The insurance plan must insure all "medically necessary" doctor and hospital services. The Act does not detail which services shall be insured, leaving this to the individual provinces and territories to decide.
3. **Universality:** All insured persons of a province or territory must have access to pubic health insurance and services on the same terms and conditions.

4. **Portability:** Provinces and territories must cover the costs of insured services for insured individuals who move or travel within Canada and when they travel outside of Canada (however, Canadians are strongly advised to purchase private health insurance whenever travelling outside the country).

5. **Accessibility:** All insured persons must have reasonable and uniform access to health services when needed, and access should not be prevented because of financial barriers or rural location. Physicians who provide insured services must be provided with "reasonable compensation."

The three criteria tied directly to the CHA's stated purpose of facilitating "reasonable access to health services without financial or other barriers" are comprehensiveness, universality, and accessibility. The public administration and portability criteria are more administrative in nature.

Provinces or territories that fail to comply with any of the five criteria may have their federal transfer payment reduced as a penalty. This is a discretionary penalty, meaning that the minister may decide whether to apply a penalty or not. The amount will be based on the seriousness of the non-compliance and will be applied as a last resort, after a consultation process that attempts to resolve the non-compliance. In general, the provinces and territories meet the requirements set out in the CHA, and many exceed them.[11] To date, no discretionary penalties have been applied.

Although the federal government plays a role in financing health care in Canada, it is the provincial and territorial governments that account for the largest source of spending on health care, as illustrated in Table 2.1.

TABLE 2.1   Provincial and Territorial Health Care Plans

Province/Territory	Health Care Plan
Alberta	Alberta Health Care Insurance Plan (AHCIP)
British Columbia	Medical Services Plan of BC (MSP)
Manitoba	Manitoba Health
New Brunswick	Medicare
Newfoundland and Labrador	Newfoundland and Labrador Medical Care Plan (MCP)
Northwest Territories	NWT Health Care Plan
Nova Scotia	Medical Services Insurance Programs (MSI)
Nunavut	Nunavut Health Care Plan (NHCP)
Ontario	Ontario Health Insurance Plan (OHIP)
Prince Edward Island	Health PEI
Quebec	Régie de l'assurance maladie du Québec (RAMQ)
Saskatchewan	Saskatchewan Health Services
Yukon	Yukon Health Care

Extra-Billing and User Charges

With the passage of the *Canada Health Act* and the change in how the federal government funded medical care, physicians could choose to **opt in** or **opt out** of the provincial health care plan. Those who opted out charged the patient for the visit and services at the point of care; in Ontario, patients were reimbursed by OHIP for the amount covered by OHIP, but not for any amount charged by the physician over and above the fee set by OHIP. Even physicians who opted in and billed OHIP directly for the visit and services provided might charge the patient an extra-billing amount at the point of care. (Many physicians were upset by the loss of fees, feeling that the amount set by provincial plans for each visit was too low. For example, a minor office visit in Ontario, for which the physician may have been charging $25 prior to the establishment of provincial medical care, was worth approximately $16 under OHIP.)

Today, all services covered under provincial/territorial health care plans must be billed directly to the government, not the patient.

Extra-billing and user charges are covered by sections 18 through 21 of the *Canada Health Act*. Although the CHA did not ban extra-billing or user charges outright, it did encourage provinces and territories to end extra-billing and user charges by subjecting those that permit these practices in respect of insured services to dollar-for-dollar federal penalties. If, for example, a province allows $1 million in extra-billing by physicians in a particular year, the federal minister of health will deduct that amount from the Canada Health Transfer for that year. The penalties are non-discretionary, meaning that the minister *must* apply them. The reason for the penalty is that the practices of extra-billing and user charges may restrict access to medical services for some Canadians for financial reasons, thereby violating the accessibility criterion.

When it was passed, the *Canada Health Act* provided that during a three-year transition period (from 1984 to 1987), any deductions in the federal contribution to a province or territory for extra-billing and user charges would be reimbursed if the charges were eliminated by the province or territory by the end of the three years. The aim of this provision was to encourage provinces to eliminate these practices. All provinces complied within the required timeframe. Penalties did not reoccur until the 1994–95 fiscal year. Today, legislation in some provinces prohibits extra-billing—for example, Ontario's *Commitment to the Future of Medicare Act, 2004*.

Role of the Public and Private Sectors in Health Care Financing and Delivery

Both the public and private sectors play important funding and delivery roles in Canada's health care system. The public sector includes federal, provincial/territorial, and municipal/local governments, and various public agencies. Most health services in Canada are paid for through health insurance plans financed by provincial governments. Governments also exert significant control over how services are delivered.

The private sector includes all non-governmental organizations and individuals, such as charities and not-for-profit organizations, as well as for-profit businesses. Hospitals and physicians fall into this category as well. The private sector is responsible for the delivery of services.

Funding

Canada's health care system is financed largely by the public sector. This includes financing by all levels of government, social security, and workers' compensation. In 2010, provincial government spending accounted for approximately 65 percent of total health expenditures (see Figure 2.1). Private sector contributions, consisting mainly of out-of-pocket expenditures by individuals for uninsured services (see the discussion below), and insurance provided by private companies accounted for approximately 30 percent of expenditures.

The federal government provides funding to the provincial and territorial governments through the Canada Health Transfer (CHT), provided they meet the criteria in the *Canada*

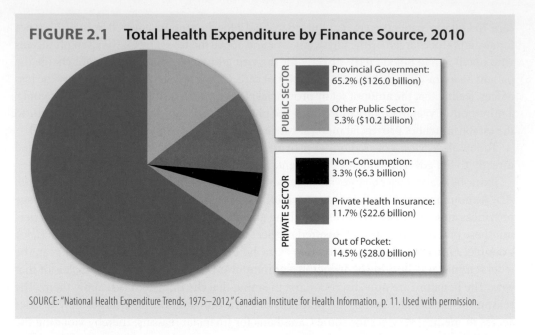

FIGURE 2.1   Total Health Expenditure by Finance Source, 2010

PUBLIC SECTOR
- Provincial Government: 65.2% ($126.0 billion)
- Other Public Sector: 5.3% ($10.2 billion)

PRIVATE SECTOR
- Non-Consumption: 3.3% ($6.3 billion)
- Private Health Insurance: 11.7% ($22.6 billion)
- Out of Pocket: 14.5% ($28.0 billion)

SOURCE: "National Health Expenditure Trends, 1975–2012," Canadian Institute for Health Information, p. 11. Used with permission.

Health Act. To address fiscal disparities among the provinces, the government also provides equalization payments to certain provinces and territories so that, regardless of their level of prosperity and their ability to raise funds through taxation, they can provide comparable public services to their residents. For example, Nunavut may not have the tax base necessary to supply appropriate health services to residents, so it may receive equalization payments to support any shortfall. The provinces and territories can use these funds to meet identified needs in targeted areas.

Public funding for health services comes from taxes levied at the federal and provincial/territorial levels. The provinces supplement these payments with other provincial revenues, such as lottery income and personal, corporate, and sales taxes. Three provinces—Alberta, British Columbia, and Ontario—charge a health premium through personal income tax. The Ontario Health Premium was introduced in 2004. It applies to individuals who are residents of Ontario and whose taxable income in a given year exceeds $20,000. The payment range's upper limit is $900.

Federal and Provincial/Territorial Roles

The federal and provincial/territorial governments share responsibility for Canada's health care system. As we have seen, the federal government is responsible for setting the national principles for the health care system under the *Canada Health Act* and providing funding to the provincial and territorial governments. In addition, under the Constitution, the federal government is responsible for providing health care services directly to certain groups of people within Canada's population. These include First Nations and Inuit, eligible veterans, inmates of federal penitentiaries, members of the Canadian Forces and the RCMP, and refugee protection claimants. The federal government is also responsible for health regulation and protection (for example, through the regulation of drugs, medical devices, and so on), health protection, consumer safety, and disease prevention. It also supports health promotion and research.

DID YOU KNOW?

The Canada Health Transfer reached $30.3 billion in 2013–14 and will reach at least $38 billion in 2018–19.

The provinces and territories are responsible for planning, organizing, and delivering health care services in hospitals and other facilities. These include home care and long-term care; mental health; all physicians' and hospital services, and services by other health care professionals; public health and health promotion initiatives; and ambulance services. Specifically, planning and organization include, for example, determining how many hospital beds will be available in a province, approving hospital budgets, determining (in consultation with the relevant bodies) which services will be insured, and negotiating fee schedules with the medical association and other health professional organizations.

Provinces also manage components of prescription care and public health services, and manage and evaluate cost-effective delivery of health services. For example, what is the optimal amount that should be allocated to health care, and what portion of the funds should be set aside for public health education, or for research and development? And, of those portions, how should funds allocated to health care be divided—for example, among preventative care, curative care, and so on?

Finally, in addition to the traditional settings of physicians' offices and hospitals, the health system includes public health, which encompasses health promotion, including mental health, sanitation, infectious diseases, and related education. Public health is the responsibility of the federal, provincial/territorial, and local/municipal governments, with the latter two shouldering most of the responsibility.

Insured, Uninsured, and De-Insured Services

Under the *Canada Health Act*, all provinces and territories are required to cover the costs of medically necessary hospital, surgical–dental, and physician services for insured persons. This usually includes access to a family doctor, emergency care, and medically necessary hospital treatment. All provinces are also required to provide medically necessary services, including acute treatment and convalescent and chronic care in approved facilities; laboratory, radiological, and other diagnostic procedures; and medically necessary emergency and outpatient services. Prescription drugs and supplies are also (usually) provided free of charge to patients in hospitals, though not outside hospitals.

The *Canada Health Act* does not specifically define what services are "medically necessary" and therefore insured. This decision is made by the provinces and territories through consultation with the appropriate medical bodies, such as colleges of physicians and surgeons (see Box 2.2). The result is that medical insurance coverage is not standard across all provinces and territories in terms of the services provided. Any service not deemed medically necessary in a particular province or territory is not insured and is paid for by the patient (through out-of-pocket expenditures, private insurance, or both).

BOX 2.2   Colleges of Physicians and Surgeons

Each province and territory has a college of physicians and surgeons. These colleges regulate the practice of medicine and work to protect and serve the public. All doctors must be members of their provincial/territorial college in order to practise medicine. The duties of the college include

- licensing physicians,
- monitoring and maintaining standards of practice, and
- investigating complaints about physicians and holding disciplinary hearings.

SOURCE: Based on data from The College of Physicians and Surgeons of Ontario.

In Ontario, insured services (see Table 2.2) are listed in the *Health Insurance Act* and in the Schedule of Benefits. In other provinces, various bodies are responsible for setting out which services are insured. For example, in British Columbia, the *Medicare Protection Act* authorizes the Medical Services Commission to set out insured services in the Medical Services Plan of BC (equivalent to the Schedule of Benefits). For any uninsured services, or when providing services to uninsured patients, physicians are permitted to charge a reasonable fee. Uninsured services in Ontario include, for example, the removal of some moles and cysts, travel immunization, the transfer of medical records, and telephone prescription renewals. As shown in Figure 2.1, private, out-of-pocket spending for uninsured services accounts for a not insignificant portion of health expenditures.

TABLE 2.2   Examples of Insured and Uninsured Services in Ontario

Insured Services	Uninsured Services
• Medically necessary physician services • Hospital services • Routine eye examinations for specified patients in specified age groups. (People 65 years and older and 20 years and younger are covered by OHIP for a routine eye examination provided by either an optometrist or physician once every 12 months plus any follow-up assessments that may be required.) • Medically necessary eye care services for patients of all ages • Dental services that require hospitalization • Limited physiotherapy services provided by designated clinics • Limited podiatry services • Insured services provided in other provinces of Canada • Services provided outside of Canada with prior ministry approval, and limited emergency services	• Services that are not medically necessary or are experimental, for example, computer-assisted surgery using telemanipulators (see eHealth section for more information) • Prescription drugs and those provided in non-hospital settings • Eyeglasses, contact lenses, refractive surgery • Routine dentistry • Cosmetic surgery that is not medically necessary

SOURCE: "Ministry Programs," Ministry of Health and Long-Term Care. © Queen's Printer for Ontario, 2008. Reproduced with permission.

This text will focus on the medical insurance that is offered under Ontario's provincial plan, OHIP. Canada's provincial and territorial health care plans are listed in Table 2.1.

In an effort to reduce public health care costs, provinces and territories de-insured a number of services in the 1990s; this has led to gaps in coverage among health services across the country. For example, routine circumcision of newborns was de-insured in Newfoundland, Prince Edward Island, Nova Scotia, New Brunswick, Ontario, Alberta, and the Yukon. Second ultrasounds in uncomplicated pregnancies were de-insured in Nova Scotia and British Columbia.[12] At the time of writing, Quebec is the only province to cover in vitro fertilization (the province covers three rounds; in Ontario, treatment is insured only in very limited circumstances).

Supplementary health services, such as prescription costs, and dental, hearing, and vision care costs, are financed privately, for the most part. Publicly funded coverage is available in most provinces and territories for individuals in certain categories, such as low-income residents and seniors. Individuals who do not qualify for these additional benefits or have other (private) coverage must pay at the point of service. Individuals may choose to purchase private health insurance from a third party, or they may be covered through a plan offered by their employers. Many employers provide medical insurance packages that cover the costs of prescription drugs and other services that are not covered by provincial/territorial health plans, such as physiotherapy, eye exams, and dental care, to varying degrees. To cover health care costs associated with injuries sustained by workers on the job, every province and territory has an employer-funded workers' compensation agency, such as the Workplace Safety and Insurance Board (WSIB) in Ontario.

OHIP

In this section, we will look more closely at Ontario's provincial health plan, the Ontario Health Insurance Plan (OHIP). The plans in other provinces and territories are set up and operate in a similar way.

OHIP dates from 1972, when hospital and physicians' services were combined under a single insurance plan. (Recall that these had been introduced at different times, following the passage of federal legislation. In Ontario, insured hospital services were introduced in 1959, and insured physicians' services were introduced in 1966.) The Ministry of Health and Long-Term Care (MOHLTC) is responsible for health care in the province. According to its website, it

> is working to establish a patient-focused, results-driven, integrated and sustainable publicly funded health system [through] helping people stay healthy, delivering good care when people need it, and protecting the health system for future generations.[13]

The MOHLTC has recently shifted its focus, becoming less involved in the actual delivery of health care and instead adopting a stewardship mandate—that is, focusing on planning and management. Specifically, it will establish the overall strategic direction and priorities for the health system and develop legislation, regulations, and policies to support these; monitor and report on health system performance in Ontario and on Ontarians' health; and develop and establish funding models for the system.

The MOHLTC is also responsible for investigating activities prohibited by Ontario's *Commitment to the Future of Medicare Act, 2004* (CFMA). Anyone (including a corporation) who contravenes the Act may be subject to the fines set out therein. The CFMA was passed to ensure that the principles of free and equitable access to medically necessary services outlined in the *Canada Health Act* are upheld in the province. To this end, it prohibits a range of practices, including the following:

- extra-billing (that is, charging more than the amount payable for an insured service under OHIP)
- charging for insured services
- queue jumping and failure to report queue jumping (that is, no one is permitted to pay or accept a payment/benefit in exchange for providing preferred access to insured services to a patient)
- inappropriate use of block or annual fees

Block fees, or annual fees, are permitted if they do not cover insured services, are applied for a specified time, list the uninsured services that they cover, and specify that payment is voluntary. Health care providers may not refuse to provide insured services because a patient refuses to pay a block or an annual fee.

SCENARIO 2.1

Dr. Nuthal charges a block fee of $150 per patient per year to patients who would like their prescriptions renewed over the phone. If a patient does not wish to pay this block fee, then he or she must make an appointment to have a prescription renewed.

Is this policy an appropriate use of the block fee? Explain.

In Ontario, as with the rest of the provinces and territories in Canada, insured services are all those covered under the *Canada Health Act*, which are medically necessary hospital, surgical–dental, and physician services. Uninsured services are listed in section 24 of regulation 552 under the *Health Insurance Act*. Ontarians pay directly for uninsured services, or these may be covered by private insurance.

Table 2.2 lists examples of insured and uninsured services under Ontario's insurance plan.

Residents of Ontario must meet certain criteria to be eligible for coverage under OHIP. An individual must (1) be a Canadian citizen, permanent resident, or among one of the newcomer-to-Canada groups who are eligible under the *Health Insurance Act*; (2) be physically present in Ontario for 153 days in any 12-month period; (3) be physically present in Ontario for at least 153 days of the first 183 days immediately after establishing residency in the province; and (4) make Ontario his or her primary place of residence.

As described above, certain groups receive coverage from the federal government and so are not eligible for provincial insurance (for example, members of the Canadian Armed Forces, RCMP, Aboriginal people, and federal penitentiary inmates).

OHIP coverage becomes effective three months after the date when an individual establishes residency in Ontario; new and returning residents should purchase private health insurance to avoid incurring costs during the waiting period. Individuals moving to Ontario from another province or territory in Canada are covered under their original provincial/territorial plan during the waiting period.

PRACTICE TIP

A new resident to Ontario may not be aware of the criteria when applying for an OHIP card. It is a good idea to have the following link on hand so that you are able to assist new residents in applying for their OHIP card: www.health.gov.on.ca/en/public/programs/ohip.

Health Care Settings and Programs

This section of the chapter reviews the main health care settings in Canada—hospitals, long-term care, home and community care, and physicians—through which care is provided, as well as related programs.

Hospitals

In Ontario, hospitals fall into four categories:

- private, not-for-profit (sometimes referred to as "public") hospitals
- private, for-profit hospitals
- federal hospitals
- Cancer Care Ontario hospitals

The majority of Canadian hospitals are private, not-for-profit hospitals over which the provincial government exerts a fair amount of authority. For example, most provincial governments set budgets for hospitals and review significant decisions of the board involving finances. The day-to-day operations of hospitals (for example, administration, laboratory, planning, and patient care) are managed by boards. Hospitals must also abide by the relevant provincial regulations and any government-mandated policies. For example, in Ontario, hospitals must observe the requirements set out in the *Public Hospitals Act*, as well as the policies set by the MOHLTC regulating the services hospitals provide. (Local health integrated networks [LHINs] will be discussed later in this chapter.)

In contrast to public hospitals, private hospitals are for-profit institutions. In Ontario today, seven private hospitals are currently operating, six of which receive funding for their operations from the MOHLTC. One example, the Shouldice Hospital just outside of Toronto, specializes in hernia surgery. In 1973, when Ontario moved to public, not-for-profit medicine, the province passed the *Private Hospitals Act*. Article 3(1) of the Act specifies that hospitals whose licences were issued before October 29, 1973 would be allowed to continue to stay in existence, but no new private hospitals could be established.[14]

Federal hospitals are owned by a department or agency of the federal government and are also run as not-for-profit institutions. Examples of federal hospitals are Veterans Affairs, Health Canada, National Defence, and Solicitor General Canada.

Cancer Care Ontario hospitals may be a separate institution but are usually areas within an existing not-for-profit hospital dedicated to caring for patients with cancer. The provincial agency that advises the government on cancer treatment is Cancer Care Ontario. This agency directs public health care dollars directly to hospitals and other cancer care institutions that deliver cancer services. There are 13 regional cancer programs in Ontario.

Long-Term Care

Long-term care facilities are typically municipal nursing homes for the aged or charitable nursing homes for the aged. Some long-term care facilities offer respite care or short-stay care. This may be provided for an individual whose caregiver is on holiday or taking a break, or for someone who is recovering from an illness or surgery whose needs cannot be met by a combination of home and community care. Long-term care homes are funded by the MOHLTC and governed by legislated standards.

The provincial government passed the *Long-Term Care Statute Law Amendment Act, 1993* (Bill 101) effective July 1, 1993, which amended the different legislation governing long-term care facilities. It brought long-term care facilities under one administrative structure within the MOHLTC. This provided consistent operational standards and consistent resident admission criteria, as well as a single funding scheme for all long-term care facilities.

Home and Community Care

Home (or community) care has become an important part of Canada's health care system. An increase in bed closures, earlier release from hospital and day surgeries, and long wait lists for long-term care have increased the demand for in-home care. **Community care access centres (CCACs)** offer many options that may help individuals stay in their homes longer. Some of these options are nursing, personal support, physical and occupational therapies, nutritional support (Meals on Wheels), and medical supplies and equipment. It is important to note that anyone can make a referral to a CCAC—the individual seeking the care, a family member, a caregiver, a friend, the individual's physician, or another health care professional.

Physicians

Physicians must have a medical degree, be licensed by the Medical Council of Ontario, and also have completed a set period of post-graduate training or residency. This is a period of two years for those applying to family practice and four to five years for those applying to a specialty practice, depending on the specialty. In Ontario, British Columbia, and Alberta, a family physician must also be certified by the College of Family Physicians of Canada. This latter period differs only in Quebec, where five to six years are required. A family physician must also be a Canadian citizen or permanent resident.

Public Health Units

Public health units (PHUs) are agencies established by municipalities to promote health and disease prevention. Each of Ontario's 36 PHUs is administered by a medical officer of health who reports to a board under the *Health Protection and Promotion Act*. Qualified staff deliver programs in schools and other organizations that promote health and disease prevention, covering such topics as healthy lifestyles, sexual health, vaccinations, addictions, growth and development, parenting education, and screening services.

In collaboration with the MOHLTC, PHUs also administer Health Smiles Ontario, a provincially funded dental program that provides basic treatment and prevention for children aged 17 and under from low-income families.

Levels of Medical Care

The three levels of medical care in the health care system are primary, secondary, and tertiary. They are illustrated and explained in Table 2.3.

TABLE 2.3   Levels of Medical Care

Primary	Secondary	Tertiary
• First point of care	• Second point of care (not usually the first point of care for the patient)	• Third point of care (in some cases may be second point of care)
• A primary care visit is referred to as an *encounter*	• A secondary care visit is usually referred to as a *consultation*	
• Provided by a health care practitioner	• Need a referral from primary health care provider	• Usually provided in a hospital setting, as the patient needs advanced medical investigation and treatment
• Primary care providers will refer a patient to a specialist (secondary care) if medical concern is beyond their scope of practice	• Provided by medical specialists	• Care provided to manage more complicated health issues, such as angina, cardiac disease, cancer, diabetes
Examples • General practitioner, family doctor • Keeping healthy people healthy, e.g., immunizations	*Examples* • Physical therapist, cardiologist, obstetrician, gynecologist • Care provided to halt or slow progress after the patient has contracted a disease or illness and has been diagnosed	*Examples* • Surgeries, cancer treatment, dialysis

These levels may overlap—that is, a patient's needs may require access to care from a combination of two or even all three levels. For example, if a patient is suffering from lower back pain, her **primary care** provider may prescribe anti-inflammatories and a referral to a physiotherapist (**secondary care** provider) to relieve the symptoms. After several visits to the physiotherapist, an MRI (magnetic resonance imaging) scan may be ordered to obtain more information at the site of pain. If the results of the MRI suggest, for example, a slipped disc, the patient's primary care provider may refer her to an orthopedic surgeon, an individual with a high level of expertise and access to a hospital (**tertiary care** provider), to have a disc repaired. Communication among all providers continues until the patient's chronic pain is resolved or can be managed at a reasonable level.

Family Practice Models, LHINs, and Compensation

Family physicians in Ontario may choose from various practice models in setting up their practice or working with others in a group practice. Different compensation models are associated with each practice model. These are outlined below.

An MA should be knowledgeable about developments in health care for several reasons: to provide patients with accurate information about how their clinic model operates, to provide information of alternative models of care so that each patient is able to make an informed decision when choosing a clinic model, and to ensure that chart documentation and billing protocol are accurate for the clinic model.

In the early 2000s, family health organizations in Ontario, the Ministry of Health and Long-Term Care, and the Ontario Medical Association (OMA) worked to develop family practice models that supported comprehensive care, health promotion, and disease prevention, treatment, and management. Services provided by a family health organization depend upon the needs of the patient population served and the size and composition of the provider team. These family health organizations are responsible for providing primary care services to their patient populations.

The discussion of family practice models refers to two terms: "enrollment" and "rostering." It is important to understand these two terms before continuing with a discussion of family practice models.

- **Enrollment:** Patients will be asked to sign a Patient Enrollment and Consent to Release Personal Health Information form upon joining many of the family practice models. They may enroll with a single family physician or with a group. On signing an enrollment form, patients agree to go to their family doctor or group first when in need of medical treatment, allow the ministry to share personal health information with their physicians or family practice model group, and not to change physicians or family practice groups more than twice per year.

- **Rostering:** Patients are required to register with a family physician or group. The rostering agreement may be informal or formal (formal agreement has both the patient and the physician signing the agreement and acknowledging their obligations to each other). Patient rostering allows the family practice, the province, and the federal government to track patient demographics. For example, once patients are rostered in a family practice, the MA will be able to describe accurately the makeup of the practice—for instance, 80 percent general, 12 percent pediatric, and 8 percent geriatric. This breakdown becomes important if the physician chooses capitation or a blended funding compensation model.

The benefits of both enrolling and rostering to a family practice or group are as follows:

- access to primary health care or advice 24 hours a day, 7 days a week
- more effective chronic disease management
- funding focused on the needs of the patient and not on the number of patients seen by the physician
- assistance for the physician or group with sharing and gathering of data for research, providing optimal care, and evaluating the practice's performance
- improvements in the MA's ability to access information needed for referrals to other health care providers, such as specialists

PRACTICE TIP

When starting as an MA for a family practitioner, take the time to learn how your physician is compensated. Research or ask questions so you fully understand the compensation model, as it may affect the way in which you register patients in the electronic health record.

Family Practice Models

The following family practice models have been developed in recent years in an effort to improve on the access to and quality of Canada's health care system, and to ensure its long-term sustainability.[15]

Comprehensive Care Model (CC Model)

This model works best for family physicians in solo practice. While patients are encouraged to enroll, this is not mandatory. The CC model offers only three hours per week outside of regular operating hours. Physicians are compensated mainly by fee-for-service (FFS) remuneration (see the section "Compensation Models," below). However, they may receive incentives or bonuses for services to any enrolled patients.

Family Health Groups (FHGs)

FHGs are very similar in design to the CC model. The major differences are that there are three or more physicians in the group (offices may be situated in separate locations but should be within reasonable proximity, that is, in the same city) and that the group must provide three to five three-hour sessions per week of patient care outside of regular office hours. Physicians are compensated the same way as in the CC model.

Family Health Teams (FHTs)

FHTs are organized like FHGs; however, the team may be interdisciplinary. It may consist of physicians, a nurse, a massage therapist, a dietician, and other health care professionals. Each team is set up based on local health and community needs. FHTs focus on providing a wider range of services, centralized care, and facilitation of communications with other health care providers. For example, FHTs may collaborate with other health care organizations, such as public health units or the Victorian Order of Nurses (VON), to meet patient needs. The FHTs are organized by local health integration networks (LHINs; see below). Physicians practising within an FHT are compensated using either a blended capitation model, complement-based base remuneration plus bonuses and incentives, or blended salary model (see "Compensation Models").

Family Health Networks (FHNs)

FHNs are organized in the same manner as family health teams. They are, however, allowed to apply to the MOHLTC for funding to recruit allied health professionals to their network. Physicians belonging to an FHN are paid using the blended capitation model but are allowed to receive fees for rostering and new patients. Physicians who provide services—such as chronic disease management, preventive care, and pre-natal care—receive bonuses, premiums, and special payments. For example, if an area is experiencing a flu epidemic, an FHN physician might receive a bonus for immunizing 90 percent of his or her practice.

Rural–Northern Physician Group Agreements (RNPGAs)

RNPGAs are family health teams but provide rural and northern communities with health care services. Typically, they involve a group of from one to seven physicians who will offer from one to five three-hour sessions per week of office hours outside of regular office hours. In addition, an RNPGA may apply to the ministry for funding to recruit allied health professionals. Physicians in an RNPGA are compensated using a complement-based remuneration model plus bonuses and incentives (see "Compensation Models").

Community Health Centres (CHCs)

CHCs are interdisciplinary teams serving communities and populations that may find it difficult to access health services otherwise. The CHC focuses on lifestyle or situational factors that can affect people's health, such as illiteracy and poor nutrition. A CHC offers both regular and extended hours, but there are no set conditions for the length and number of extended office hours. Physicians are employed by the CHC and receive a fixed salary.

Local Health Integration Networks (LHINs)

The *Local Health System Integration Act, 2006* created **local health integration networks (LHINs)** in Ontario to promote a more patient-centred health care system that strives to put an end to communities' providing health care in isolation, by offering integrated health care services. There are 14 not-for-profit LHINs across the province. Each LHIN is responsible for planning, coordinating, integrating, funding, and evaluating the delivery of health care services in its area. LHINs do not deliver health care services but promote and help develop partnerships among physicians, hospitals, access centres, community support services, community mental health and addictions services, community health centres, and long-term care facilities. To develop each LHIN, people in their communities—the general public, patients, advocates, and health services professionals—were consulted. Then a plan was tailored to local needs and priorities, drawing on the resources listed above, that would meet provincial strategic directions. The hope was that the community's needs would be met locally and that patients would not have to seek help great distances away.

Compensation Models

The MOHLTC and the OMA have developed several compensation models. Many of these models are based on blended payments—a model may be predominantly one form of payment, plus financial incentives or bonuses. In most physician offices, the MA is responsible for completing the billing, and it is his or her responsibility to understand the different models of compensation and to provide the government with the correct forms and information to ensure that the physician is paid. Two terms used when discussing compensation models are "fee-for-service remuneration" and "capitation."

In the **fee-for-service remuneration** model, health care professionals receive a fee (or payment) for each patient seen and service provided. Total remuneration is based on the number of patients seen and the type of visit. For example, most physician appointments are booked at 15-minute intervals, and each of those intervals would be billed under an A001A code (minor assessment) and be valued at $22.30. So if the physician were able to see 30 patients that day, the base remuneration for that day would be $669. The service must be approved by OHIP. The Schedule of Benefits (see Chapter 9, "Medical Billing") lays out the remuneration received for each service. The number and description of services is sent to OHIP on the 18th of every month (except December, when the remittance date is the 15th). OHIP deposits the remuneration amount directly into the physician's business bank account in the month following the submission.

Capitation is another payment method used by health care insurance services (e.g., OHIP) to remunerate physicians. The physician is paid a contracted rate regardless of the number of patient visits within each month. The payment amount is determined on the basis of the demographics of each practice (that is, age, sex, illness, and regional differences). For example, a physician with a high percentage of geriatric patients may receive a higher monthly amount than one who sees a higher percentage of 20- to 50-year-olds. It is assumed that the practice with a higher number of geriatric patients will experience more patient visits.

The following are types of capitation compensation models:

- **Blended capitation model:** Physicians receive a base payment per patient. However, each physician is also able to receive incentives and special payments for the provision of specific primary health care services. The base payment amount is calculated by taking the physician's enrollment and multiplying it by the capitation rate.
- **Complement-based base remuneration:** Compensation is based on the number of physicians within the group and their commitment to offering regular and reasonable extended office hours. This compensation model offers a base remuneration plus funding to meet overhead costs accrued in managing the services within the community.
- **Blended salary model:** Physicians are salaried employees of an organization or community-sponsored family health team, and their salary is based on the number of patients rostered to each individual physician within the team. Bonuses and special payments may be achieved through the provision of specific primary health care services, for example, ensuring that every patient on the physician's roster has an up-to-date immunization record.
- **Salaried model:** The physician's salary is based on the patient population. Physicians are salaried employees of community health centres that provide care to a specific patient population.

Developments in Health Care

New family practice models, changes to physician remuneration, and electronic health technologies, such as electronic health records and telehealth, are important motivators of innovation, sustainability, and efficiency in our health care system today. Improving health care delivery, patient safety, quality of care, and productivity, and implementing the use of electronic health records, will streamline the process of delivering health care in Canada and facilitate the integration of services across health care providers. The primary developments are in the area of eHealth, telehealth, and patient safety.

eHealth and Telehealth

eHealth

In 2008, the provincial government established eHealth Ontario to address how information and communication technologies are being used in health care. A goal of eHealth is to help physicians and other health care providers establish and maintain **electronic health records (EHRs)**—the sharing of necessary medical information among health care providers. The application of eHealth is demonstrated in hospital settings, home care, and physicians' offices. eHealth enables electronic patient administration and **telemedicine**, which includes *teleconsultations*, *telepathology*, and *teledermatology*, as well as monitoring of vital signs, diabetes, asthma, and home dialysis. An experimental aspect of telemedicine is computer-assisted surgery using *telemanipulators*, in which a robotic arm carries an endoscope while two other manipulator arms carry interchangeable tools, such as scissors and grippers. Just as important, but perhaps more mundane, eHealth also provides a medium for health awareness and education.

The most commonly known eHealth technology is the electronic health record. Telemedicine allows physicians to use information technology to provide medical care and diagnostic services to patients from a distance through digital transmission of voice, images, and data rather than through a face-to-face visit. With the development of digital technology and IT, such as desk cams, digital imaging, and picture archiving, physicians are able to integrate telemedicine into the EHR. "The key," says Dr. Sarah Muttitt of the Canadian Society of Telehealth, "is to integrate telemedicine with the key health care issues facing the system today such as waiting-list management, chronic disease management and public health."[16]

Telemedicine is usually thought of when trying to bring medical care to rural and isolated communities; however, many of these communities may not have the infrastructure to support the technology (see Table 2.4). Canada Health Infoway states that "an estimated 15 percent of Canada's rural or remote communities have telemedicine coverage of some kind, such as videoconferencing facilities. According to 2003 figures from Health Canada, about 34 telemedicine provider networks covered 895 sites across the country."[17]

TABLE 2.4   Barriers to and Advantages of Telemedicine

Despite the advantages, there are many barriers to telemedicine that need to be overcome.

Barriers	Advantages
How to pay physicians for their time	Better access to health care
Issues of jurisdiction and licensure for physicians	No wait list or loss in travel time
How to provide the infrastructure needed for rural communities to access services	Productivity—physicians are able to treat more patients
How to ensure the security of information collected	No travel costs

In 2012, five provinces/territories—Yukon, Quebec, Ontario, British Columbia, and New Brunswick—had telemedicine programs in place, called "home telehealth." Home telehealth allows a physician to monitor a patient's medical condition from that patient's home. The patient is able to monitor vital signs, such as pulse, blood pressure, blood sugar, and weight, and send the data directly to the physician for review. Most assessments take only minutes and eliminate the need for the patient to travel to and from the physician's office. Another benefit of home telehealth is that the physician has a record of the patient's results over a long period of time rather than just from a weekly or monthly office visit.

There are several barriers to the complete acceptance of telemedicine. However, Canada needs to develop new health care delivery models to meet the increasing demand. Programs such as telemedicine and other eHealth initiatives may be the key to providing high-quality care and equal access for all patients in each of Canada's provinces and territories.

Telehealth Ontario

Telehealth Ontario provides free, quick and easy, bilingual access to a qualified health professional (a registered nurse) who is able to assess your symptoms and provide guidance on whether to care for yourself, see your family doctor, or head straight to the emergency department.

Telehealth provides an alternative to heading the emergency department or family physician's office as the first point of care. The nurse is available for advice 24 hours a day, 7 days a week. It is important to note that Telehealth does not replace 911—always call 911 in an emergency.

Patient Safety

Ensuring the safety of every patient utilizing health care services is a concern and an important challenge to Canada's health care system. Patient safety—reducing medical errors or adverse events—is the main focus of Canada's efforts to improve the quality of care provided across the system. The federal, provincial, and territorial governments are working together with health care providers to continue to develop and implement plans to eliminate risk factors in the delivery of health care.

Some Challenges Facing Canada's Health Care System

There are a number of concerns today regarding the future of the Canadian health care system. These fall into the general categories of cost, quality of care, and wait times.

Cost

According to the Conference Board of Canada, our health care system is facing a financial crisis: "Without change to the structure of Canada's health system, public health care expenditures will increase from 31 cents of every provincial and territorial tax dollar in 2000 to 42 cents by 2020."[18]

Our aging population and the need for increasingly costly technology are placing a monetary strain on the health care system. As people retire and the working population shrinks, the dollar amounts through taxes that may be funnelled into paying for health care decrease. If health care funding diminishes, then support for our aging population is at risk. Many elderly people may be forced into retirement homes or long-term care facilities, unable to maintain their independence, which in turn would burden the current health care system. Although new primary health care delivery methods have been developed (for example, FHTs and LHINs) and are improving overall care, Ontario will have to continue to explore information technology and become more innovative at providing affordable and efficient health care to patients. The costs of maintaining the privacy of personal information contained and transmitted in electronic health records is another area of concern.

The provinces and territories face some common challenges in managing the rising cost of health care—aging populations, shrinking tax base, growing debt. The white paper *Measuring What Matters: The Cost vs. Values in Health Care*[19] suggests that our health care system move toward a system focused on strengthening health and the quality of life for Canadians, look at how health care is delivered, and focus on health and wellness rather than illness.

Quality of Care and Wait Times

Another concern for Ontarians has been the quality of their health care. The *Excellent Care for All Act*, passed in 2010, was developed to help improve patient care and introduced annual public quality improvement plans for every hospital. The Act linked hospital executive compensation to achievement of quality improvement targets and put in place a number of requirements for hospitals, including mandatory public reporting on nine key patient safety indicators (*Clostridium difficile* infection, hand hygiene compliance, surgical site infection, and other measures); patient and employee satisfaction surveys; and a patient complaints process. As well, it created Health Quality Ontario (HQO), an agency responsible for promoting evidence-based standards of care and recommending best practices for all those in the health care system.

Reducing wait times has been a goal in Ontario since 2004. While the government has had some success in reducing wait times for key health services, such as hip and knee replacements, cardiac procedures, surgeries, and MRI and CT (computed tomography) scans, these health services are granted at the referral of a specialist, and the wait time to see a specialist is still too long. All provinces now monitor and publish wait times; Ontario publishes this information on the MOHLTC website. The Canadian Institute of Health Information (CIHI) also provides wait-time data. Ontario's wait times are better than those of most Canadian provinces but well below international standards.

Finding better solutions to care for an aging population, improving the quality of care, and reducing wait times are all required to ensure that Canada's health care system remains viable and is able to meet the needs of patients.

NOTES

1. Canadian Museum of Civilization, http://www.civilization.ca/cmc/exhibitions/hist/medicare/medic-1h03e.shtml.

2. Canadian Museum of Civilization, http://www.civilization.ca/cmc/exhibitions/hist/medicare/medic-1h11e.shtml.

3. Canadian Museum of Civilization, http://www.civilization.ca/cmc/exhibitions/hist/medicare/medic-1h06e.shtml.

4. Canadian Museum of Civilization, http://www.civilization.ca/cmc/exhibitions/hist/medicare/medic-1h15e.shtml.

5. Canadian Museum of Civilization, http://www.historymuseum.ca/cmc/exhibitions/hist/medicare/medic-2h01e.shtml; and Douglas–Coldwell Foundation. (n.d.), http://www.dcf.ca/en/tommy_douglas.htm.

6. Canadian Broadcasting Corporation, http://www.cbc.ca/history/EPISCONTENTSE1EP14CH3PA5LE.html.

7. Canadian Museum of Civilization, http://www.historymuseum.ca/cmc/exhibitions/hist/medicare/medic-5h02e.shtml.

8. Parliament of Canada, http://www.parl.gc.ca/content/sen/committee/371/soci/rep/repintmar01part1-e.htm.

9. Health Canada, http://www.hc-sc.gc.ca/hcs-sss/pubs/system-regime/2011-hcs-sss/index-eng.php.

10. Ibid.

11. Health Canada, http://www.hc-sc.gc.ca/hcs-sss/pubs/cha-lcs/2012-cha-lcs-ar-ra/index-eng.php.

12. Madore (2005), http://www.parl.gc.ca/content/lop/researchpublications/944-e.htm - btheroletxt.

13. Ministry of Health and Long-Term Care, http://www.health.gov.on.ca/en/ministry/default.aspx.

14. *Private Hospitals Act*, RSO 1990, c. P.24, s. 3(1), http://www.e-laws.gov.on.ca/html/statutes/english/elaws_statutes_90p24_e.htm.

15. For more information on these models and the means of remuneration for physicians working in them, see HealthForceOntario, http://www.healthforceontario.ca/en/Home/Physicians/Training_|_Practising_Outside_Ontario/Physician_Roles/Family_Practice_Models.

16. "Telemedicine: Ready for Prime Time?," http://www.facturation.net/multimedia/CMA/Content_Images/Inside_cma/WhatWePublish/LeadershipSeries/English/telemedicine.pdf.

17. Ibid.

18. Conference Board of Canada, http://www.conferenceboard.ca/e-library/abstract.aspx?did=59.

19. Snowdon et al. (2012), http://sites.ivey.ca/healthinnovation/files/2012/11/White-Paper-Measuring-What-Matters.pdf.

RESOURCES

Health Council of Canada:
    http://www.healthcanada.gc.ca

REFERENCES

Boychuk, G.W. (2012). Grey zones: Emerging issues at the boundaries of the *Canada Health Act*. Commentary no. 348. Toronto: C.D. Howe Institute. http://cdhowe.org/pdf/Comm_348.pdf.

Canadian Museum of Civilization. (2010). *Making Medicare: The history of health care in Canada, 1914–2007*. http://www.civilization.ca/cmc/exhibitions/hist/medicare/medic01e.shtml.

Health Canada. (2004). Federal role in health. http://www.hc-sc.gc.ca/hcs-sss/delivery-prestation/fedrole/index-eng.php#a1.

Health Canada. (2012). *Canada Health Act: Annual report, 2011–2012*. http://www.hc-sc.gc.ca/hcs-sss/pubs/cha-lcs/2012-cha-lcs-ar-ra/index-eng.php.

Health Canada. (2012). Canada's health care system. http://www.hc-sc.gc.ca/hcs-sss/pubs/system-regime/2011-hcs-sss/index-eng.php.

Madore, O. (rev. 2005). The *Canada Health Act*: Overview and options. http://www.parl.gc.ca/Content/LOP/ResearchPublications/944-e.htm.

Makarenko, J. (2010). Canada's health care system: An overview of public and private participation. http://mapleleafweb.com/features/canada-s-health-care-system-overview-public-and-private-participation.

Ministry of Health and Long-Term Care (MOHLTC). (2008). Protecting access to public health care. http://www.health.gov.on.ca/en/public/programs/ohip/cfma.aspx.

Snowdon, A., Schnarr, K., Hussein, A., & Alessi, C. (2012). *Measuring what matters: The cost vs. values of health care*. White paper. Ivey International Centre for Health Innovation. London, ON: Western University. http://sites.ivey.ca/healthinnovation/files/2012/11/White-Paper-Measuring-What-Matters.pdf.

uOttawa. (2009). Health care policy in Canada. http://www.med.uottawa.ca/sim/data/Health_care_policy_milestones_e.htm.

REVIEW QUESTIONS

True or False?

1. A health care system is strictly composed of physicians and hospitals.

2. Private, for-profit hospitals in Ontario are not licensed by the Ministry of Health and Long-Term Care.

3. The federal government subsidizes the provinces through income tax placed on the Canadian taxpayer.

4. Today, a patient is charged at the point of service.

5. Canada's provincial health insurance is publicly funded.

6. The principal federal organization overseeing health care is Health and Welfare Canada.

7. The *Long-Term Care Statute Law Amendment Act* was passed in 1993.

Fill in the Blank

1. Name the four types of hospitals found in Ontario: _____, _____, _____, and _____.

2. The BNA Act stands for the _____ Act.

3. Upset with capitation (fee-for-service remuneration), physicians were initially allowed to _____ of the billing structure presented by the *Canada Health Act*.

4. Some services are not funded by provincial health insurance plans because they are not medically _____.

5. The three levels of medical care are _____, _____, and _____.

Multiple Choice

1. The federal government is responsible for the health care of all but ONE of the following:
   a. Inuit
   b. veterans
   c. First Nations
   d. government officials

2. Each provincial government is responsible for its
   a. hospitals, physicians' services, public health, home care, long-term care, mental health services, and ambulance services
   b. hospitals, public health, home care, long-term care, mental health services, and ambulance services
   c. hospitals, physicians' services, public health, home care, long-term care, and mental health services
   d. hospitals, physicians' services, home care, long-term care, mental health services, and ambulance services.

3. The following services are considered basic and must be included in all provincial insurance plans:
   a. acute treatment, convalescent and chronic care, and most laboratory and diagnostic procedures
   b. convalescent and chronic care, most laboratory and diagnostic procedures, and plastic surgery
   c. acute treatment, convalescent and chronic care, most diagnostic procedures, and eye exams
   d. acute treatment, driver physicals, chronic care, and most laboratory and diagnostic procedures

4. To receive coverage from OHIP, you must be a Canadian citizen and have lived in Ontario for a minimum of
   a. 6 weeks
   b. 6 months
   c. 3 months
   d. 3 weeks

5. Which one of the following is a new development in family practice?
   a. public health units
   b. long-term care facilities
   c. home care
   d. family health networks

Short Answer

1. Name the two legislative acts that had the most influence on the Canadian health care system.

2. Which groups receive medical coverage from the federal government but not the province or territory?

3. Name and define the three levels of health care.

4. How does a family physician receive remuneration?

5. What criteria provide proof of eligibility to receive medical insurance?

6. Name and describe two developments in family health practice.

7. List five insured and five uninsured OHIP services.

HYBRID LEARNING

Using Blackboard's online discussion board, provide a response to the following questions in paragraph form using 200–300 words.

1. Search for "Health Council of Canada Progress Report 2013: Health Care Renewal in Canada" and locate the report. Read either the section on disease prevention, health promotion, and public health or the section on Aboriginal health. Post your thoughts on how the country has done in attempting to achieve the 2004 10-year plan for the section you chose.

2. Comment on at least two of your classmates' posts. Comments must be substantial and not just "like," "agree," "disagree," etc.

3. Read the two articles below.
   - "Why Our Health Care System Works for Canada," by Robert McMurtry, *The Globe and Mail*, March 24, 2014.
   - "The Future of Medicare: Three Possible Scenarios," by Martin Zelder, *BC Medical Journal, 42*(5), June 2000.

   Consider the following questions and post your answer to *one* of the questions on the Blackboard discussion board. *Link* your answer to one of the articles.

   a. Do you agree that Canadians are blessed? Why or why not?

   b. Should health care in Canada be government funded, or should Canadians help through taxation to cover health care costs? Explain.

   c. Do you believe that the Canadian health care system is fair and effective? Explain.

ACTIVITIES

1. Research your local integrated health network (LIHN). What services does it offer? Is its location easily accessible? What total population does it serve?

2. Compare the Canadian and Australian health care systems.

3. Create your own timeline for the development of health care in Canada. Your timeline must have between five and ten significant dates or events. Why do you feel these dates/events are significant?

4. Match the abbreviation with the correct meaning.

   Meanings

   1 *Canada Health Act*
   2 *British North America Act*
   3 Ontario Health Insurance Plan
   4 Canadian Medical Association
   5 Canada Health Transfer
   6 Ministry of Health and Long-Term Care
   7 Health Quality Ontario

   Abbreviations

   A BNA Act
   B HQO
   C CMA
   D OHIP
   E MOHLTC
   F CHT
   G CHA

5. Match the definition with the term.

   Definitions

   1 Responsible for health care in the province of Ontario
   2 Determined the responsibilities of each level of government at the time of Confederation
   3 Amount paid by the federal government under the *Federal–Provincial Fiscal Arrangements and Established Programs Financing Act*
   4 Health care insurance plan for the province of Ontario
   5 An agency responsible for promoting evidence-based standards of care and recommending best practices for all those in the health care system
   6 A national organization that provides leadership to Canadian physicians, and advocates for access to high-quality health care
   7 Combines the *Hospital Insurance and Diagnostic Services Act and the Medical Care Act*

   Terms

   A Health Quality Ontario
   B Canadian Medical Association
   C *Canada Health Act*
   D Ministry of Health and Long-Term Care
   E Canada Health Transfer
   F *British North America Act*
   G Ontario Health Insurance Plan

The Medical Office Environment

3

LEARNING OUTCOMES

After completing this chapter, you should be able to:

- understand workplace health and safety legislation and the standards in a medical office
- define ergonomics and explain how it influences employee productivity and prevents injury
- identify the features of an efficient workstation and office layout, including lighting and the modular office
- understand the principles of inventory control
- understand the importance of a procedure and policy manual, and create one for your workplace
- outline procedures for maintaining the medical office
- identify procedures for maintaining office security

> The supreme quality for leadership is unquestionably
> integrity. Without it, no real success is possible, no
> matter whether it is on a section gang, a football field,
> in an army, or in an office.
>
> —Dwight D. Eisenhower

Introduction

The concept of "workplace" is broad and encompasses many factors. In addition to the physical location, it includes a number of variables, such as workstation and office setup, temperature control, air quality, noise, physical aesthetics, safety, workload, child care, and parking—to name just a few.

In recent decades, workplace health and safety has come to the forefront in many countries, including Canada. Provincial and territorial legislation provides workers with basic rights and places duties on employers with which they must comply. The aim is to ensure that all workers can enjoy a safe workplace in which they are protected against injury and that supports their long-term physical and mental health and well-being. In addition to complying with legislative provisions, a well-designed workplace enhances productivity, efficiency, and job satisfaction. This chapter will look at all these topics. The main areas of a medical office, and the specific requirements for each, will be examined. We will also describe the specific duties of the MA with respect to controlling inventory and ordering supplies, the office procedure and policy manual, and office security.

Occupational Health and Safety

DID YOU KNOW?

Various organizations across Canada provide recommendations on workplace health and safety practices. Additional information on the topics covered in this chapter is available from the Canadian Centre for Occupational Health and Safety, the Ministry of Labour, and the Industrial Accident Prevention Association.

In Canada, every workplace is regulated by either the federal or the provincial/territorial government and has a legal duty to meet the requirements of occupational health and safety legislation. Health professionals, including physicians, are regulated by the provincial government. In Ontario, the applicable legislation is the *Occupational Health and Safety Act* (OHSA), which was passed in 1979.

The OHSA sets out the rights and duties of all parties in the workplace. Its primary purpose is to protect workers from work-related health and safety hazards. The Act outlines procedures for dealing with hazards, and provides penalties for failing to comply with its provisions. Under section 66, the maximum penalty for an individual failing to comply with the OHSA or its regulations is a fine of up to $25,000, up to 12 months' imprisonment, or both; for a corporation, the fine is up to $500,000.

An important component of the Act is the internal responsibility system (IRS). The IRS gives every person in an organization, regardless of his or her position, direct responsibility for health and safety. The intention is that everyone take the initiative on health and safety issues and contribute to improving safety on an ongoing basis, both individually and with others in the workplace.

Rights and Duties of Workers

Under the OHSA, all workers have the following three rights:

1. The *right to know* about any hazards in their workplace to which they may be exposed, and what to do about them. The requirements of the Workplace Hazardous Materials Information System (WHMIS)—which is a Canada-wide system designed to provide information about hazardous materials used in the workplace to employers and employees—are an important example.

2. The *right to participate* in identifying and solving health and safety problems. This right is expressed mainly in the requirement for a joint health and safety committee (JHSC) and a worker representative on the committee.

3. The *right to refuse work* that they believe is unsafe.

In addition to the rights above, workers also have a duty to take responsibility for their personal health and safety. This means they should not behave in a way that would endanger others or themselves. Section 28 of the OHSA lists some specific duties of workers. Workers must do the following:

- Work in compliance with the OHSA and its regulations, and follow the policies and procedures in place in their workplace.
- Use any equipment, protective devices, or clothing required by the employer.
- Tell the employer about any missing or defective equipment/protective device that may be dangerous.
- Report any known workplace hazard or violation of the OHSA to the employer.

Examples of guidelines that employees in a medical office setting may be required to follow include:

- Close file drawers when not in use and open only one file drawer at a time.
- Clear paths and entrances of snow and ice.
- Clean up spills immediately.
- Alert the employer if carpeting is not fixed securely to the floor or is not in good repair.
- Avoid cables crossing pedestrian routes where possible.
- Use a stepladder or other appropriate ladder to reach heights, not a chair or anything on wheels.
- Do not overload electrical circuits; use appropriate extension cords.
- Provide sufficient lighting both indoors and outdoors.
- Lock up all valuable personal items such as purses and wallets.
- Keep emergency telephone numbers accessible near the phone.
- Be familiar with emergency procedures, such as what to do in case of a fire, a bomb, a medical emergency, or any threat of violence.
- Follow safety precautions in using all office equipment.

Duties of the Employer

Sections 25 and 26 of the OHSA place general and specific duties on employers. In general, employers must do everything reasonable in the circumstances to protect the health and safety of their workers; ensure that all equipment, materials, and protective equipment are in good working order; provide employees (and their supervisors) with information, instruction, and supervision to make sure they know how to work safely and are able to do so; and cooperate with the JHSC.

Specifically, employers must comply with the OHSA and its regulations, develop and implement a health and safety program and policy, post a copy of the OHSA in the workplace, and provide health and safety reports to the JHSC.

Violence and Harassment in the Workplace

Employees have a right to work in an environment in which they feel safe. A toxic environment that includes abusive or hostile behaviour—whether by the employer, other employees, or customers or clients—can have negative effects on employees' mental and physical well-being, and can affect employees' commitment to their work and their productivity.

In 2010, changes aimed at strengthening protections against workplace violence and addressing workplace harassment came into effect in Ontario. The changes were the result of Bill 168, and they apply to all workplaces covered by the OHSA.

The OHSA now includes a definition of "workplace violence."[1] It means:

- the exercise of physical force by a person against a worker, in a workplace, that causes or could cause physical injury to the worker
- an attempt to exercise physical force against a worker, in a workplace, that could cause physical injury to the worker
- a statement or behaviour that it is reasonable for a worker to interpret as a threat to exercise physical force against the worker, in a workplace, that could cause physical injury to the worker

Violence or the threat of violence may be introduced into a workplace by a number of individuals, including workers, supervisors, and managers; intimate partners, family members, or friends; students; patients or clients; and strangers with no ties to the workplace.

The OHSA also defines "workplace harassment." Workplace harassment means engaging in a course of vexatious comment or conduct (that is, behaviour that tends to cause annoyance, frustration, or worry) against a worker in a workplace that is known or ought reasonably to be known to be unwelcome. This may include, but is not limited to, bullying, threats, intimidations, degrading comments, offensive jokes or innuendos, displaying or circulating offensive pictures or materials, or making offensive or intimidating phone calls.

The Canadian Centre for Occupational Health and Safety provides the following examples of workplace bullying:[2]

- spreading malicious rumours, gossip, or innuendo that is not true
- excluding or isolating someone socially
- intimidating a person
- undermining or deliberately impeding a person's work
- constantly changing work guidelines

- establishing impossible deadlines that will set up the individual to fail
- intruding on a person's privacy by pestering, spying, or stalking
- assigning unreasonable duties or workload that are unfavourable to one person
- underwork—creating a feeling of uselessness
- yelling or using profanity
- criticizing a person persistently or constantly
- belittling a person's opinions
- blocking applications for training, leave, or promotion
- tampering with a person's personal belongings or work equipment

The effects of harassment can range from mild to severe and may include feelings of frustration, helplessness, anxiety, or anger; loss of confidence; physical symptoms such as loss of appetite, problems with sleep, stomach pains, or headaches; difficulty concentrating; and decreased productivity and morale.

Under the OHSA, employers have an obligation to implement workplace violence and harassment policies that include details on how to file a complaint alleging harassment or violence, and what steps the employer will take when a complaint is filed; procedures for obtaining assistance immediately in the event of workplace violence or violence that is likely to occur; and controlling identified risks.

BOX 3.1 Workplace Bullying DOs and DON'Ts

If you feel that you are being bullied, discriminated against, victimized, or subjected to any form of harassment:

DO

- FIRMLY tell the person that his or her behaviour is not acceptable and ask them to stop. You can ask a supervisor or union member to be with you when you approach the person.

- KEEP a factual journal or diary of daily events. Record:
  - The date, time, and what happened in as much detail as possible
  - The names of witnesses
  - The outcome of the event

  Remember, it is not just the character of the incidents, but the number, frequency, and especially the pattern that can reveal the bullying or harassment.

- KEEP copies of any correspondence (e.g., letters, memos, emails, faxes, texts) received from the person. Save any voicemail messages.

- REPORT the harassment to the person identified in your workplace policy, your supervisor, or a delegated manager. If your concerns are minimized, proceed to the next level of management.

DON'T

- DON'T retaliate. You may end up looking like the perpetrator and will most certainly cause confusion for those responsible for evaluating and responding to the situation.

- DON'T accept or endure bullying or harassment. You deserve to be treated professionally and work in a safe environment.

SOURCE: Reproduced from "Bullying in the Workplace," Canadian Centre for Occupational Health and Safety. Used with permission.

Even if a workplace does not have a program in place, employees still have the legal rights outlined here, and the employer still has a duty to investigate the employee's concerns and make an effort to fix the unlawful behaviour. If there is no program in place, employees should send a formal memo to the employer or human resources department outlining what has occurred and asking the employer to investigate and intervene. If the employer fails to do so, the employee will have further grounds for legal action that may need to be taken in the future.

Workers who believe they are in danger from workplace violence have the right to refuse work, and reprisals by the employer are prohibited. The provisions also place a duty on employers, who are aware or ought reasonably to be aware that domestic violence may spill over into the workplace, to take every reasonable precaution to protect workers at risk.

Note that in the small number of cases that end up in court, the courts will evaluate the conduct objectively—not every workplace stress that an employee complains of will be found to have violated the law.

Office Setup and Ergonomics

First impressions are important, and in the case of a health care setting, play a significant role in helping patients feel at ease as soon as they enter the office. Patients' first impression should be that the office is clean and well organized and that the ambience is welcoming, friendly, and warm, while still being professional. The physical environment can foster a feeling of confidence, on the part of patients, in the medical care they are about to receive.

In addition to giving a professional appearance, it is important that the office be designed in a way that maximizes efficient workflow and supports the health of employees. In this section, we will examine the factors involved in creating the ideal medical office environment for patients and staff.

The Main Areas in a Medical Office

Each area of a medical office serves a different function, and the setup recommendations below are tied directly to its purpose. In addition, the CMA has published a useful module titled *Setting Up Your Medical or Clinical Office*, which includes detailed checklists of each area in the physician's office. To view this resource, visit the CMA's website and search for Module 15.

The Reception Area

The reception area of a medical office should welcome patients. Ideally, it is not a waiting area, but a place for patients to be greeted, checked in, and ushered to the waiting area.

The focus of the reception area is the desk, and it should be easily located as soon as the patient enters the physician's office. The reception area should be located far enough away from the waiting area so that when patients check in, they do not feel that everyone waiting is able to hear any personal details they share with the MA or receptionist (see Figure 3.1).

The Waiting Area

This area should consider patients' comfort and privacy. Because wait times may be long, the waiting area should provide ample seating so that no one is left standing while waiting for an appointment. The design and furniture in the waiting area should allow patients of all sizes to be easily accommodated. For example, chairs without arms accommodate larger patients more easily. Also, choose chairs over sofas or couches. Couches are usually harder to keep clean, and many patients consider this type of seating too intimate.

PRACTICE TIP

First impressions include a patient's impression of personnel. Make sure that you greet patients cordially and with a smile.

FIGURE 3.1

The Reception Area

This reception area and waiting room allow for very little privacy. The glass partitions help protect phone conversations, but leave patients checking in or out vulnerable to having private or personal information overheard by other patients in the waiting room.

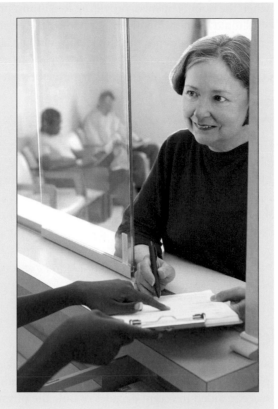

SOURCE: Stockbyte/Thinkstock.

The office administrator often has enough influence to place his or her stamp on the atmosphere created in the waiting area. A waiting area should be designed to invite patients in, not to add stress to their day. There are several inexpensive ways to ensure that a waiting area is more welcoming and comforting to patients. For example, choose artwork for the walls that is peaceful, portraying non-violent themes; add a few green plants, and play relaxing music (instrumental music is preferable to music with words) at a volume just below conversational level. Good music to try is "new age" or classical, or music composed specifically for relaxation. The added benefit of relaxation music, especially in a small office, is that it will provide more privacy for conversations occurring at the reception area.

The waiting area should be bright and provide up-to-date educational and entertaining reading material, such as general-interest magazines. Wall colours should be cheerful, and surfaces should be easy to clean. A carpeted waiting area will absorb more noise, will keep the room quieter, and will contribute to a more soothing, less clinical atmosphere. However, carpet can be challenging to keep clean. Providing child-sized chairs or tables (if space allows), with books (e.g., picture books, activity books), small toys, and games, will make the wait much easier for patients with children.

The Exam Area

A model exam room design considers patient and physician interaction, privacy, efficiency, and accessibility. Exam rooms should be large enough to comfortably accommodate the physician, the patient, and at least one family member. There should be seating available for the family member, and the space should be wheelchair accessible. The room should include a sink, exam table, desk, supplies, and a storage space for these and other required equipment. There should also be extra chairs, as well as room on one wall for a sharps container.

To ensure privacy, the exam room should ideally be soundproof. The door should swing inward, into the room, not outward; this prevents the inside of the room being visible to the waiting room when the door is opened, providing maximum privacy for the patient inside. Each exam room should be multifunctional, providing the opportunity for it to be used for more than one purpose. For example, the physician should be able to record patient history, perform a Pap test or a small surgical procedure (e.g., wart removal), or provide family counselling in the same exam room. This will help reduce wait times.

SCENARIO 3.1

You were hired by a family physician six weeks ago. You are enjoying the new job, and everyone is friendly and welcoming. When you arrived today, the waiting room was full but unusually quiet. You noticed that one of your co-workers was sitting at reception checking a patient in. She was speaking very loudly at the patient, who seemed to be hard of hearing. Unfortunately, the whole waiting area could hear what was being discussed.

Later today, there is to be a staff meeting consisting of the physician, nurse, and support staff. You feel that the situation in the morning compromised confidentiality. Will you address it at the staff meeting? Why or why not? How would you suggest the office handle the issue?

Ergonomics

Chapter 1 discussed psychological stress and the toll it can take if unaddressed. This chapter deals with physical self-care—especially, prevention of injuries.

Awareness has expanded in recent decades of how the physical conditions of our work and our workspaces affect our physical health on a daily basis and over time. Our bodies allow us to carry out everyday tasks, but sometimes the way we use or position them can put strain on our muscles and joints. If uncorrected, these stressors can cause serious injuries called **musculoskeletal disorders (MSDs)**. The areas most commonly affected by MSDs are the back, shoulders, neck, elbow, hands, and wrists. Symptoms include pain, tenderness and swelling, stiffness or reduced range of motion, and numbness or tingling.

Ergonomics is the study of the relationship between humans and their work environment—specifically, how we interact with and are affected by our workplace and its component parts. Ergonomics includes physical factors, such as office furniture, equipment, and workstation setup, and environmental factors, such as lighting, temperature, and noise. All contribute to the quality of our work environment and how it affects us.

The ultimate aim of ergonomics is to provide a work environment that prevents injury and promotes productivity. Workers must be able to complete their duties in a way that contributes positively to their long-term health, without sitting or standing for too long, without straining the eyes, or remaining in awkward postures, all of which might cause **repetitive stress injuries (RSIs)**.

DID YOU KNOW?

Musculoskeletal disorders (MSDs) affect thousands of workers every year. In addition to individual pain and suffering, the associated absences and lost productivity cost Ontario's workplaces hundreds of millions of dollars annually. MSDs are the number one lost-time work injury reported to the WSIB each year.

Physical Conditions

The physical conditions in an office consist of the overall layout of the office as well as individual workstations.

Office Layout

Office layout refers to the organization and arrangement of equipment and furniture within a given area of floor space. A well-designed office layout contributes to a pleasant, space-efficient, and safe office. A good design assists workflow, allows for proper space utilization, facilitates change, and creates a healthy working environment.

If you, as the MA, have the opportunity to choose the office layout, consider the following while deciding how best to use the floor space:

1. *Position equipment to optimize work and traffic flow.* Place noisy equipment away from phones, but not so far that administrators have a long walk to retrieve documents. The setup should permit wheelchair and stroller access.

2. *Make full use of floor space, but leave room for growth.* The setup should be flexible enough to accommodate growth and change in the office. For example, as the physician's practice grows, you will need to add more filing cabinets for chart storage.

3. *Place the reception desk away from the waiting area.* As described above, this will help prevent people in the waiting area from overhearing discussions at the reception area.

4. *Present a welcoming and relaxing first appearance.* Keep the reception and waiting areas clean, and provide a place for patients to hang coats and leave boots. Also, remember to greet patients and other visitors with a smile.

5. *Accommodate different arrangements of furniture.* Some people like to work facing the doorway, while others will be constantly distracted if there is a window or doorway in their peripheral vision.

6. *Set up work areas or cubicles so that doorways are staggered.* This allows more privacy and less distraction.

The office layout may consist of closed offices or open modular spaces. Closed offices provide privacy from noise and interruptions, but may not create a sense of unity and the desire to work together to meet the needs of the office. Moreover, many offices may not have been built with individual closed offices. If the layout is open, consider how the desks are spaced. Is there enough space between desks, and is there a barrier that will allow each worker to have clearly defined personal space? In an open space, it is important to consider the placement of large machines, such as photocopiers. They should be accessible yet far enough away to avoid noise interruption.

The open floor plan was designed to improve communication among workers, thereby improving productivity. This type of plan also saved companies space and money. Unfortunately, the open floor plan produced unanticipated results—the loss of privacy made conversation difficult and confidentiality almost impossible. To minimize the negative effects of an open floor plan, many businesses provide "white noise" in the form of piped-in music, which makes it difficult for those in adjacent cubicles to hear each other's conversations. Despite these drawbacks, open floor plans are still the most popular, as they offer significant savings in cost.

Workstation Setup

In a medical office, the MA's workstation usually consists of a chair, desk, computer, phone, work in progress, individual files, and other office accessories. We will examine these below.

THE CHAIR

The chair is the most personal piece of office equipment. A good chair has five legs, provides lumbar support, and has the following adjustable features:

- *Seat height and seat tilt.* The seat should be set at a height that allows the feet to rest flat on the floor. This prevents pressure on the back of the legs and stress on the spine. For optimal weight distribution, the recommended seat tilt is five degrees. The seat should adjust at a variety of angles to allow for changing positions and postures for different tasks.
- *Backrest height.* The backrest must be adjustable to offer the best lumbar support. The lower end of the backrest should be positioned just above the hipbone. The backrest should allow for a slightly reclined sitting position.
- *Backrest horizontal position.* This supports the body when the individual is sitting all the way back in the chair. The thigh muscles—not the backs of the knees—must support the body weight.
- *Armrest position.* The armrest height should allow the lower arm to rest comfortably on the armrest, usually at elbow height, while the person is keying. Elbows should be kept close to the sides of the body.

Figure 3.2 shows the ideal position of various parts of the body—including the head, eyes, back, elbows, thighs, and feet—when someone is seated at a desk using a computer. You should be able to perform the necessary adjustments to your office furniture in order to achieve this setup.

FIGURE 3.2 Ideal Position for Working at a Computer

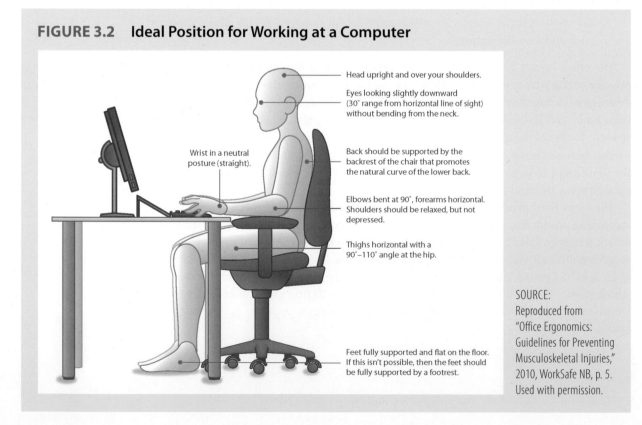

Head upright and over your shoulders.

Eyes looking slightly downward (30° range from horizontal line of sight) without bending from the neck.

Wrist in a neutral posture (straight).

Back should be supported by the backrest of the chair that promotes the natural curve of the lower back.

Elbows bent at 90°, forearms horizontal. Shoulders should be relaxed, but not depressed.

Thighs horizontal with a 90°–110° angle at the hip.

Feet fully supported and flat on the floor. If this isn't possible, then the feet should be fully supported by a footrest.

SOURCE:
Reproduced from "Office Ergonomics: Guidelines for Preventing Musculoskeletal Injuries," 2010, WorkSafe NB, p. 5. Used with permission.

BOX 3.2   Health Effects of Long-Term Sitting

In the past few years, research has shown that sitting long hours at a desk greatly affects personal health. Even moderate to vigorous activity may not offset the health risks attributed to sitting for long periods of time—cardiovascular disease, cancer, high blood pressure, and diabetes. Suggestions to minimize the effects of a sedentary job are to stand while on the phone or eating lunch, use a standing desk, or exchange your standard chair for an exercise ball. This last suggestion will not only keep your core engaged but inspire you to add a "sitting jacks" or figure-of-eights motion to break up long periods of sitting.

SOURCES: Based on "What Are the Risks of Sitting Too Much?" by James A. Levine, MD, PhD, Mayo Clinic, and "Too Much Sitting Linked to Chronic Health Problems," by Mary Elizabeth Dallas, *HealthDay News*.

As you learned in Chapter 1, when you remain in one position for a long period of time—and in particular, if you are sitting or engaged in repetitive, stationary tasks—your muscles and joints start to fatigue and your circulation decreases. Sitting at a computer in the same position for long periods causes lower back pain, neck and shoulder stiffness, and RSIs such as carpal tunnel syndrome. In the long term, a sedentary job can cause MSDs and other health conditions. To decrease the negative effects of sitting at a desk, take stretch breaks throughout the workday. Appendix 3.1 at the end of this chapter provides a series of stretches you can do at your desk.

THE DESK

The top of the desk should be at elbow height, measured while the arms are hanging relaxed at the sides, with the elbows bent at a right angle (see Figure 3.2). The height may be adjusted by raising or lowering the desk or chair. If height must be adjusted by raising the chair, you may have to use a footrest to ensure proper positioning of the feet. If you have the opportunity to choose your desk, suggest that desks be provided that can be raised or lowered to suit either standing or sitting.

Keyboard and mouse trays may be used to bring the work surface to elbow height. However, be sure there is enough space to sit with your legs tucked under your work surface.

Keep your phone and current work within easy reach. Avoid reaching behind the midline of the body, or twisting, to reach items (see Figure 3.3). If possible, use a headset or speakerphone to prevent neck injury (though, if using speakerphone, keep in mind the privacy considerations discussed earlier in this chapter; this option may not be feasible in your office).

COMPUTER, KEYBOARD, AND MOUSE

In general, the monitor should be placed at a distance of 60–90 centimetres from the eyes (see Figure 3.4). The appropriate distance will vary according to the user's eyesight and age, and the size of the monitor. The monitor should be centred in front of you, with the top of the monitor just below eye level, and tilted about 15 degrees to the back.

As described above, the elbows should be kept close to the sides of the body, with elbows bent at 90 degrees. The wrists should be straight when keying, not angled up or down, and the hands should float above the keyboard (see Figure 3.5). Various ergonomic keyboards are available to help maintain the hands in a neutral position.

The mouse should be at the same level as the keyboard, and placed within easy reach.

Environmental Conditions

Environmental conditions are another contributing factor to employee health and productivity. How do temperature, noise, lighting, and colour affect us?

PRACTICE TIP

Take charge of your health at work. Set aside two to five minutes every hour for a "micro-break": stop what you are doing, get up and walk around, stretch (see Appendix 3.1), or change to a different task. If you aren't able to leave your desk, try some stretches at your desk.

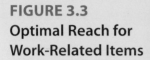

FIGURE 3.3
Optimal Reach for Work-Related Items

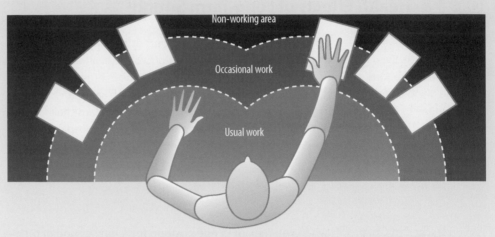

SOURCE: Reproduced from "Office Ergonomics: Guidelines for Preventing Musculoskeletal Injuries," 2010, WorkSafe NB, p. 7. Used with permission.

FIGURE 3.4   Optimal Position Relative to Monitor

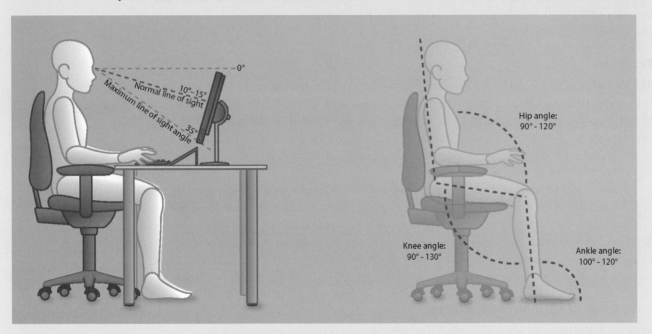

SOURCE: Reproduced from "Office Ergonomics: Guidelines for Preventing Musculoskeletal Injuries," 2010, WorkSafe NB, p. 10. Used with permission.

FIGURE 3.5   Awkward, Neutral, and Correct Wrist Postures

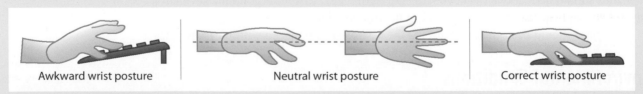

SOURCE: Reproduced from "Office Ergonomics: Guidelines for Preventing Musculoskeletal Injuries," 2010, WorkSafe NB, p. 8. Used with permission.

- *Lighting.* Apart from helping us see, the type of lighting in a space can affect our productivity and our mood. For optimal ergonomic lighting, choose more than one source of diffused or soft light. Natural light often causes glare on the computer screen, so if the monitor is located near a window you should use a screen protector to minimize eyestrain caused by glare.

- *Temperature.* Thermostats should be set to provide constant temperature within a comfort zone of 20 to 23 degrees Celsius. Temperatures that are too cold or too hot can cause discomfort and decrease productivity.

- *Noise.* Noise is often irritating and acts as a distraction. If it is loud enough and occurs for a long period of time, it may also cause health problems. To reduce noise in the office:

  - Place photocopiers at the farthest possible distance from the desk areas that still provides convenient access.

  - Choose carpet rather than tile or hardwood for floors (or, if your office does not have carpet, consider placing carpets strategically around the office), or have employees wear soft-soled shoes.

  - If the office layout is modular, choose sound-absorbing panels for the office modules.

  - Try to position office cubicles away from conference rooms, break areas, and entrances/exits.

- *Colour.* Studies have shown that colour affects how we feel. The appropriate use of colour can maximize productivity, minimize fatigue, and make one feel calm. Following are some general guidelines:

  - Intense colours, such as bright red, may contribute to feelings of anxiety.

  - "Institutional beige" and taupe are not exciting colours and don't cause any problems, but neither do they inspire creativity.

  - Cool colours (blue and green) in the right shade boost creativity, improve reading ability, and have a calming effect.

  - Warm colours (soft red and orange) boost appetite and energy, make people feel cautious and detail-oriented, and increase accuracy.

Supplies, Equipment, and Inventory Control

As an MA, you will be responsible for ordering both general office supplies and medical supplies. It is important that you implement and follow procedures to ensure that office and medical supplies are always in stock in sufficient quantities. A balance must be struck between ensuring the office has enough stock on hand so you do not run out of anything, and trying not to be overstocked. Overstocking will not only use up too much space but items may become spoiled or expire, wasting money. A well-managed inventory contributes to the efficient running of the office.

Whether you are in a new or established office, when managing supplies and equipment, the task will be easier if you separate the needs of the front and back areas.

- front areas: reception, office, and waiting area(s)
- back areas: exam rooms, bathrooms, and possibly a staff room

Supplies for the front areas include everything the MA requires to complete daily tasks, for example, paper, pens, a stapler, copier, fax machine, envelopes, filing materials, and paper

PRACTICE TIP

One person should be in charge of keeping track of inventory and ordering supplies for the office. This is usually the MA, unless there is an office manager. *All* employees should be responsible for restocking areas within the office that are running low.

clips—as well as magazines and other materials for the waiting room. Supplies for the back areas include items needed for patient care, such as needles, prescription pads, bedding, specula, thermometers, cotton balls, bandages, disposable gloves, and so on.

As an MA, it is up to you to decide on the method of inventory tracking you wish to use. In most medical offices, visual control is used. This technique is simple: you look at inventory on hand and decide whether to order more. To keep on track using this method, also use a **tickler system** to track day-to-day use. A tickler system uses master lists that are posted at supply areas. The staff check off inventory used on a daily basis, which helps the MA know when inventory is running low and when to place an order to restock (see Table 3.1).

When inventory is running low, the MA will place an order to restock the supply. To keep track of each item, the quantity kept on hand, and the ordering amounts, create a spreadsheet, as shown in Table 3.2. This spreadsheet will be kept on the computer and will act as a reference when the tickler lists show that an item needs to be ordered.

Medical supplies are ordered from various suppliers. The suppliers chosen will likely depend on the city and surrounding area of the medical office, as well as the MA's preference.

In this discussion, assume that we are controlling inventory for an established office, so we are not purchasing furniture, instruments, or equipment. Our focus is medical supplies (e.g., syringes, needles, exam paper, bandages, reagent strips, gauze, lancets, swabs, gloves, tongue depressors, Pap kits) and stationery supplies (e.g., paper, letterhead, envelopes, filing supplies, stamps, prescription pads, chart stickers). Medical and stationery lists may be kept together; however, most MAs prefer to separate the types of supplies into two lists. These lists may be simpler than the spreadsheet shown in Table 3.2. The list would need only three columns: one to itemize the supply, another for the staff member to mark amount taken, and the third to indicate original amount of the item (see Table 3.1).

> **PRACTICE TIP**
>
> Be aware of the budget allotted for stocking both the front and back offices, and keep your spending within this amount. Keeping track of inventory will also indicate any misuse or waste of supplies and whether the budget should be adjusted.

TABLE 3.1   Medical Supply Inventory Checklist

Date Inventory Created:			
Item Description	**Quantity in Stock**	**Quantity Removed**	**Initials**
Swabs	3 doz	6	AV
Tongue depressors	4 doz		
Exam table paper, 12 rolls/box	1 box	1 roll	SP
Gauze, 4x4	1 box		
Gauze, 2x2	1 box		
Syringes	1 doz		
Vaginal specula	1 box		
Gloves (assumes use of app. 20/day)	S-M-L: 3 boxes each size	1 box sm	KT
Lancets	1 box		
Tape	1 box		
Pap smear kit	2 doz		
Reagent strips, urine pregnancy	1 doz		

TABLE 3.2   Inventory Supply List

Inventory ID	Name	Description	Unit Cost	Quantity in Stock	Reorder Level (when to reorder)	Reorder Time in Days
	Vaginal specula	16				
	Ear syringes	2				
	K-basins (2)	2				
	Scalpel handles	3				
	Tissue forceps	2				
	Sponge forceps	2				
	Dressing forceps	2				
	Ear curettes	4 sizes x 1 doz each				
	2-mm punch biopsy	1 box				
	5-mm dermal curettes	1 box				
	2-mm dermal curettes	1 box				
	Nasal specula	2				
	Nasal forceps	1				
	Metzenbaum scissors	1				
	Uterine sound instrument	1				
	Thermometers, digital	2				
	Syringes 3 cc, 25 Gx 5/8" (used a lot)	1 doz				
	Syringes TB, 26 G (allergy)	1 doz				
	Scalpel blades, #15	½ box				
	Exam table paper, 12 rolls/box	1 box				
	Gauze, 4x4	1 box				
	Gauze, 2x2	1 box				
	Sigmoidoscope tubes, 25/box	1 box				
	Anoscopes, 25/box	1 box				
	Sharps containers	2				
	Tape, bandages	6				
	Reagent strips, urine GP	1 box				
	Reagent strips, urine 4 MD	1 box				
	Reagent strips, blood glucose	1 box				
	Reagent strips, urine pregnancy	1 box				
	Lancets	1 box				
	Eye patches	1 box				
	Gloves, vinyl (assumes use of app. 20/day)	S-M-L: 1 box each size				
	Tongue depressors	1 box				
	Cotton swabs	1 box				
	Personal lubricant gel	1 box				
	Cervical cytobrushes, culture medium, Pap smear kit	2 doz				
	Lidocaine, 1% and 2%	1 of each strength				

When controlling inventory, follow these basic guidelines:

1. *Know what you have.* If you do not know what you have, you may run out of an item or duplicate an item. Both are costly mistakes.

2. *Keep track of how fast you use supplies.* This information will provide you with a guide as to how much you use over a given period. Then, you will be able to order the correct amount. You should aim to place an inventory order once a month. Therefore, stock shelves so that all items last for an equal amount of time. You do not want to have to order a different supply each week.

3. *Keep an inventory list in the storeroom and a duplicate list on a computer spreadsheet.* The list in the storeroom will allow staff to fill in supplies used on a daily basis, which can then be transferred to the computer spreadsheet for reference when ordering.

4. *Organize stock with shelf and drawer labels.* This will allow easy and quick locating and restocking of supplies.

Reordering medical supplies is much easier if you are aware of items that need to be reordered. Whenever possible, use a purchase order (PO) to place your supply order. If this is not possible, be sure to keep a written record of the order to avoid mistakes and disagreements with suppliers. A PO or written record will also provide you with a cross-reference against the supplier's packing slip. Always compare the packing slip to the actual inventory shipped by the supplier when the order arrives. Check off everything that is received, and make a note of any missing items, back-ordered items, or discrepancies on the packing slip. Place new stock on the shelf as soon as possible.

Procedure and Policy Manual

A **procedure and policy manual** is a written guide describing office routines and practices. It may also include additional information, such as contact numbers and sample forms. Whether the MA needs to know how to book a patient, open a new chart, or complete required health forms, a procedure and policy manual will offer an overview of the steps involved.

"Procedure" and "policy" mean two different things. "Procedure" establishes processes and how to complete them, and "policy" establishes the rules. For example, a procedure could give step-by-step instructions on how to open the clinic for the day, and a policy would state that the office doors are never opened earlier than 8:45 a.m. In addition, as an ongoing point of reference for all staff, the manual can be used to orient new employees and to guide temporary workers through various daily tasks.

For a procedure manual to be easy to use, it must be clear and easy to read and provide simple, step-by-step instructions on how to complete each task. Procedure and policy manuals vary in size and content, depending on the type of information they contain. Most manuals are housed in a three-ring binder so that they can be updated easily through the simple addition or removal of pages. The manual should be formatted in a consistent manner, and will include headings, subheadings, and screen shots to help the reader understand the material.

The office procedures manual should be detailed and contain an easy-to-use index, a table of contents, or both. It may also use tabs to help users find information quickly and easily. It should contain examples or samples of forms, both blank and filled in, and checklists to guide office staff through various procedures, such as opening and closing the office and daily tasks. For a sample daily office routine, see Box 3.3.

PRACTICE TIP

A clear and well-organized supply list will allow anyone who is covering for you when you are away to continue your usual ordering and stocking procedures easily, without interruption.

PRACTICE TIP

All employees should have access to the procedure and policy manual. The manual acts as a reference guide for duties and responsibilities, as well as a guide to the proper completion of forms (including templates), billing, and other office procedures. New or temporary employees should be given the procedure manual and instructed to review it.

While the specific content of the manual may vary among offices, there are a few areas that are consistently covered: a mission statement; greeting and patient registration; job descriptions; chart setup and management; filing; communications procedures, including mail, telephone, and email procedures; billing; supply management; patient preparation; stocking of exam rooms; office security; emergency procedures; referrals; staff list and contact information; and office dress code.

BOX 3.3   Sample Daily Office Routines

The following list of tasks may appear in a procedure and policy manual:

Opening

- Unlock door
- Disable alarm
- Turn on lights
- Adjust the heat/air conditioner to a comfortable temperature
- Make sure patient charts are pulled for today's appointments
- Ensure that all rooms are open and ready for patients
- Check phone messages
- Check email
- Replenish the paper in all printers
- Tidy up waiting room while on the way to unlock the front door at 8:00 a.m.

Daily

- Check mail
- Prepare the examination rooms for the next patient
- Continuously check email for incoming correspondence
- Empty OUT baskets

Closing

- Check examining rooms; restock supplies
- Pull charts for the next day
- Set phones to "night answer"
- Turn off lights
- Set alarm
- Lock door

Let's review some of the manual contents in more detail:

- *Mission statement.* A mission statement describes the goals and purpose of the medical office. For example: "To provide comprehensive, high-quality medical care in an efficient and caring environment."

- *Job descriptions.* These should present detailed responsibilities for each job category within the office, with the exception of the physician.

- *Chart setup.* New or temporary MAs must be able to open a new patient file. To do this, they will need instructions detailing file folders and labels used, what information is needed to open a new client file on the database, and how each file label is set up.

- *Filing.* New or temporary MAs need to know what type of filing system is used, where files are stored, what to do when a file is removed from the office (charge-out system), and how files are managed throughout the day. For example, a procedure and policy manual might specify the following:

  - File by last name, first name, in alphabetical order.

  - Files are organized according to patients treated in the last five years, inactive files five years and over, and deceased patients.

  - Patient's files that have been accessed throughout the day must be returned to the proper location in the file room at the end of every day. This practice will help reduce the risk of lost patient records.

  - All patient records for the day's appointments will be pulled in the morning to guarantee ease of use throughout the day.

  - When removing a file, insert a pink sign-out slip with the date, time, and your name to maintain security of patient records. Only a physician should remove files from the office. An MA may take a chart to work on it only while at the office.

  - If you are not sure how the filing system works, ask another office member to ensure that you are following the proper filing procedures.

- *Telephone procedures.* New or temporary MAs must be provided with information on how to answer the phone, the hours during which the phone is answered, message-taking criteria, how to page physicians, and how to deal with inter-office calls and long-distance calls. For example, a procedure and policy manual might specify the following:

  - Remember to smile when speaking on the phone. This automatically makes you sound genuine and friendly toward the person on the other end of the line.

  - Answer the telephone on or before the third ring.

  - Greet all callers with a friendly salutation, such as "good morning" or "good afternoon," state your name, state the name of the medical office, and ask how you may help them.

  - If you are working with a patient in the office and the phone rings, politely excuse yourself for a moment, answer the telephone, and ask the caller if he or she would mind being placed on hold. If the caller agrees to be placed on hold, press the HOLD button, and then gently hang up the phone. Don't forget that you have a caller on hold!

  - Be sure to record all messages. Messages should contain callers' first and last names, phone number, the reason for the call, and date and time of call.

  - If the message is regarding a patient, the message slip should be attached to the patient's chart before handing the message to the physician.

  - Be sure to check the voicemail system frequently.

  - When making a callback to a patient wishing to book an appointment, make sure that you are logged in to the EMR and that your Scheduler tab is selected. Be sure to inform the patient that you are calling from the medical office and that you are returning his or her call.

  - If you are calling a patient with information from the physician, follow the steps above and be sure to have the physician's notes in front of you before you call.

- *Mail, patient greeting, and registration.* New or temporary MAs must be provided with information on how to handle incoming and outgoing mail, proper greetings, and how to register a patient. For example, with regard to mail, a procedure and policy manual would contain instructions on procedures as to where and when the mail is

PRACTICE TIP

Remember that as an MA, you are not permitted to provide any medical advice whatsoever. Advise callers who are in an emergency situation to hang up immediately and dial 911.

delivered or collected, how to sort the mail and what to do with sorted mail, and procedures for outgoing mail. With regard to patient greeting and registration, the manual might specify the following:

- Greet each patient with a smile and welcome him or her to the office.

- Mark the patient's arrival on the day sheet and/or in the EMR.

- Have new patients complete a New Patient Form, located in the top drawer of the smallest filing cabinet behind the reception desk.

- Ask the patient for his or her health card, and record the number and version code.

- Have the patient take a seat until the doctor or nurse is ready to see him or her.

- When a patient is finished with the appointment and is checking out, be sure to book any follow-up appointments indicated by the physician.

- If diagnostic testing or referrals are required, inform the patient that he or she will receive a call within 10 days with the information regarding the appointment.

SCENARIO 3.2

You picked up the mail and began to open and sort it. As you are examining a piece of mail, you realize that you have accidentally opened an envelope marked "Personal and Confidential." What do you do?

Office Security

Medical offices are opportune places for theft or vandalism because of the drugs that are often kept on the premises and the expensive equipment they may contain. As an MA, it is your responsibility to ensure that every precaution is taken to secure the premises. All staff members should receive instruction on office security measures and be able to set and disable the alarm. The MA is often responsible for doing this.

A list detailing the office protocol for security should be kept on hand. The following is a sample:

- Minimize the number of prescription pads, and keep extras stored in a secure place. This will prevent a patient, staff member, or other person from taking a pad and attempting to forge a prescription.

- Lock filing cabinets and cupboards containing medical records, drugs, or cash.

- Keep track of keys that have been distributed to employees, cleaning staff, and others. Make sure that individuals who are no longer employed by the practice return their keys. If there are two entrances, do not use a single master key for both doors.

- Install an alarm system, and change the alarm code frequently.

- Do not leave the reception area unattended. Make sure that someone (you or another staff member) is always present.

- Make patients and other office visitors aware of the fact that you have a security system. This can be as simple as posting the stickers provided by the alarm company.

- When the office is closed, make sure that the answering machine is turned on. If you use an answering service, let them know that you have closed the office for the day.

- For computer security, ensure that IT has installed firewalls.

- Shut down or disconnect computers and routers at the end of the day.

- Password-protect all computer log-ins.

NOTES

1. "Definitions," http://www.labour.gov.on.ca/english/hs/sawo/pubs/fs_workplaceviolence.php.

2. "Bullying in the Workplace," http://www.ccohs.ca/oshanswers/psychosocial/bullying.html.

RESOURCES

Canadian Centre for Occupational Health and Safety:
   http://www.ccohs.ca

Ministry of Labour (Ontario):
   http://www.labour.gov.on.ca

Industrial Accident Prevention Association:
   http://www.iapa.ca

Canadian Medical Association:
   http://www.cma.ca

McKesson Supply Manager Overview Video:
   http://www.mckesson.com

REVIEW QUESTIONS

True or False?

1. Ergonomics looks only at the office layout.

2. One way to prevent injury or fatigue is to take a three-minute activity break every day.

3. Phone headsets are not considered useful in the medical office setting.

4. A medical office procedure manual is used only by new employees.

5. A packing slip includes items on backorder.

6. Every employee should have access to the procedure manual.

7. The *Occupational Health and Safety Act* was passed in 1979.

Fill in the Blank

1. A _____ gives the MA guidelines and resources to complete the daily tasks in a medical office.

2. Two functions of the reception area are _____ and _____.

3. A spreadsheet would be commonly used for _____.

4. Over time, strain on muscles and joints can cause _____ disorders.

5. The office security alarm code should be changed _____.

6. The *Occupational Health and Safety Act* established _____ rights of workers.

Multiple Choice

1. An important consideration when deciding how to position the computer monitor at the reception desk is
   a. patient confidentiality
   b. lighting
   c. staff access
   d. position of the printer

2. When a shipment of supplies is received, the shipment should be checked against the
   a. advertised prices
   b. enclosed packing slip
   c. invoice
   d. requisition slip

3. Which of the following might cause a repetitive stress injury?
   a. an overworked employee
   b. fumes from cleaning agent spillage
   c. exposure to electromagnetic radiation
   d. a workstation that does not include ergonomic furniture

4. Which of the following should be included in a section of the office policy manual?
   a. confidentiality
   b. job description
   c. opening procedures
   d. all of the above

5. To ensure that the medical office has the supplies it needs, the medical administrator should establish a(n)

   a. inventory log

   b. reorder point

   c. order quantity

   d. all of the above

6. Which of the following does NOT contribute to office ergonomics?

   a filing cabinets

   b. lighting

   c. desk chair

   d. paint colour

7. Which of the following would NOT be found in the reception area of a medical office?

   a. something to keep children busy

   b. five-legged desk chair

   c. office resources

   d. a headset

8. Environmental ergonomics does NOT refer to

   a. lighting

   b. air quality

   c. desk size

   d. noise

Short Answer

1. Define ergonomics.

2. List five guidelines for office safety.

3. Explain the purpose of a procedure and policy manual.

4. Why is the role of the receptionist so important in putting the patient at ease?

5. Explain why inventory records are kept.

6. As a new employee, where would you look to find your own or a co-worker's job description, if you needed to refer to it in the course of your work?

HYBRID LEARNING

1. Watch the first 44 seconds of the McKesson Supply Manager Overview Video. Then, on the McKesson website, go to Providers, Physicians, Medical–Surgical Supplies and Services, Technology Solutions. Finally, answer the following questions:

   a. What, if any, are the benefits of a web-based ordering system?

   b. Identify three ways in which you are able to locate products.

   c. Would you recommend a web-based ordering system for your office? Explain.

2. Environmental allergies and/or sensitivities, such as mould, perfumes, latex, off-gassing from paints, solvents, and so on, have become a very big concern in the workplace today. Using an Internet search (see the links in Appendix 3.2 at the end of this chapter), research the following:

   a. Are carpets still considered safe flooring in the workplace?

   b. Why are most workplaces "scent free"?

   c. What are some of the risks of working in an environment with mould?

   d. What does "off-gassing" mean?

3. Search for and find the Canadian Centre for Occupational Health and Safety sample checklist for offices. Look at the following areas of the Office Inspection Checklist on the next page: General, Material Storage, Lighting, Equipment, and Floors.

   a. Think of your family doctor's office, or visit the health centre of an administrative office on campus, and complete the table on the next page.

   b. Were you surprised by your inspection? Explain.

OFFICE INSPECTION CHECKLIST			
Location:		Date:	
Answer the following questions. You may answer **Y** (Yes) or **N** (No), where appropriate.			
Flooring	What is the floor covering?		
	Is there loose material, debris, worn carpeting?		
	Are the floors slippery, oily, or wet?		
Equipment	Are guards, screens, and sound-dampening devices in place and effective?		
	Is the furniture safe?	Worn or badly designed chairs	
		Sharp edges on desks and cabinets	
		Poor ergonomics (keyboard elevation, chair adjustment)	
		Crowding	
	Are ladders safe and well maintained?		
Lighting	Are lamp reflectors clean?		
	Are bulbs missing?		
	Are any areas dark?		
Material Storage	Are materials neatly and safely piled?		
	Are there stepladders or stools to get to materials on higher shelves?		
	Are storage shelves overloaded or beyond their rated capacity?		
	Are large and heavy objects stored on lower shelves?		
	Are passageways and work areas clear of obstructions?		
General	Are extension cords used extensively?		
	Are electrical or telephone cords exposed in areas where employees walk?		
	Are machines properly guarded?		
	Is electrical wiring properly concealed?		
	Does any equipment have sharp metal projections?		
	Are wall and ceiling fixtures fastened securely?		
	Are paper and waste properly disposed of?		
	Are desk and file drawers kept closed when not in use?		
	Are office accessories in secure places?		
	Are materials stacked on desks or cabinets?		
	Are file cabinet drawers overloaded?		
	Are file cabinets loaded with the heaviest items in the bottom drawers?		
	Are filing stools or wastebaskets placed where they might be tripping hazards?		

ACTIVITIES

1. Create an office layout floor plan that demonstrates ergonomic principles to avoid on-the-job injury.

2. **a.** Using the inventory list in Table 3.1 as a reference for amounts of stock, organize the storeroom. Use the following table to list each stock item on the appropriate shelf.

STOREROOM INVENTORY		
Shelf	*Item*	*Reason*
Top Shelf		
Shelf 3		
Shelf 2		
Bottom Shelf		

STOCK ITEMS

- ☐ 5" Dressing Forceps
- ☐ Adhesive Fabric Bandages—Knuckle
- ☐ Adhesive Plastic Bandages
- ☐ Adhesive Plastic Bandages, 1" Diameter Spot
- ☐ Alcohol Prep Pads
- ☐ Antiseptic Cleaners
- ☐ Bathroom Tissue
- ☐ Cotton-tipped Applicators
- ☐ Diagnostic Penlight

- ☐ Disposable Drapes, Fanfold
- ☐ Dri-Sorb Underpads
- ☐ Elastic Bandages
- ☐ Examination Paper
- ☐ Gauze Sponges
- ☐ Halsted Mosquito Forceps
- ☐ Iodine Swabs
- ☐ Non-woven Sponges, Sterile
- ☐ Powder-free Synthetic Exam Gloves

- ☐ Pregnancy Test Strips
- ☐ Single-fold Towels
- ☐ Specula
- ☐ Steri-Strip Skin Closures
- ☐ Tenaculum Forceps
- ☐ Tissues
- ☐ Various Replacement Bulbs (e.g., exam lights, laryngoscopes, ophthalmoscopes)
- ☐ Waxed Paper Cups

b. What features should be added to the shelves to make the storeroom even easier to navigate and to help keep it organized?

c. Explain why you placed certain items where you did. (For example, where will you place items that are potentially hazardous, and why? Where might you place large, bulky items, and why?)

APPENDIX 3.1

Computer and Desk Stretches

Sitting at a computer for long periods often causes neck and shoulder stiffness and, occasionally, lower back pain. Do these stretches every hour or so throughout the day, or whenever you feel stiff. Photocopy this and keep it in a drawer. Also, be sure to get up and walk around the office whenever you think of it. You'll feel better!

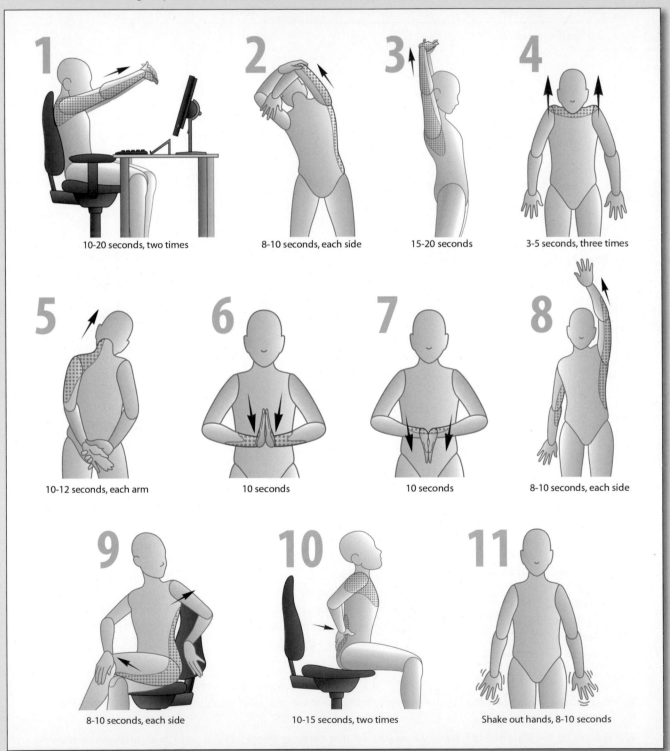

1 — 10-20 seconds, two times

2 — 8-10 seconds, each side

3 — 15-20 seconds

4 — 3-5 seconds, three times

5 — 10-12 seconds, each arm

6 — 10 seconds

7 — 10 seconds

8 — 8-10 seconds, each side

9 — 8-10 seconds, each side

10 — 10-15 seconds, two times

11 — Shake out hands, 8-10 seconds

SOURCE: Reproduced from "Office Ergonomics: Guidelines for Preventing Musculoskeletal Injuries," 2010, WorkSafe NB, p. 13. Used with permission.

APPENDIX 3.2
Web Links

SEDENTARY LIFESTYLE RISKS

- http://www.ncbi.nlm.nih.gov/pmc/articles/PMC2996155/
- http://www.mayoclinic.org/healthy-living/adult-health/expert-answers/sitting/faq-20058005
- http://apps.washingtonpost.com/g/page/national/the-health-hazards-of-sitting/750/

ENVIRONMENTAL HEALTH HAZARDS

- http://www.ccohs.ca/oshanswers/hsprograms/scent_free.html
- http://www.cdc.gov/niosh/topics/indoorenv/chemicalsodors.html
- http://www.cdc.gov/niosh/topics/indoorenv/mold.html
- http://www.ccohs.ca/oshanswers/biol_hazards/iaq_mold.html

Medical Records 1: Legal Framework and Requirements

4

LEARNING OUTCOMES

After completing this chapter, you should be able to:

- explain the importance of maintaining accurate and up-to-date medical records
- identify the legislation and the regulatory guidelines that govern medical records in Ontario
- understand the importance of keeping patients' personal information confidential
- identify concerns and proper practices related to technology, phone calls, and communication, working with records, and storing records in a medical office setting
- outline when consent is required and when it is not, with respect to the collection, use, and disclosure of patients' personal information
- explain the rules for storing, transferring, retaining, and destroying patient records in Ontario

> W*hat use is knowledge if there is no understanding?*
>
> —Stobaeus

Introduction

Every time a patient sees a physician, a record is made. **Medical records**, or charts, tell the story of a patient's health, and they are essential to physicians and any other health care professionals involved in treating a patient.

Physicians have many legal and professional obligations with respect to medical records, and helping to ensure these are met is an important part of your work as an MA. Medical records must be maintained accurately, and the information they contain must be kept confidential and secure in accordance with various provincial and territorial legislation and regulatory guidelines.

Complete and up-to-date records enable physicians to provide patients with the highest quality of care. Records are also used by others in the patient's health care team—that is, the other doctors and specialists, as well as the hospitals, pharmacies, and laboratories, involved in the care and treatment of a patient (sometimes called the "circle of care").

DID YOU KNOW?

The value of documenting an individual health record has been recognized for centuries. The earliest evidence of documenting health care records can be seen in ancient cave writings. Over the years, the documentation and maintenance of medical records have evolved through cave writing, clay tablets, hieroglyphics, papyrus, paper, and now electronic files.

It is important to note that the patient record is a *legal document*, and that the appropriate provincial licensing body or ministry of health may review it at any time. Because charts demonstrate the quality and continuity of care, they are an important source of evidence in any investigation where the care provided by a physician is in question—for example, in civil, criminal, or administrative matters and in inquiries made by the Office of the Chief Coroner or the College of Physicians and Surgeons of Ontario.

An inadequate health care record threatens the quality of health care and may lead to medication errors, prolonged recovery, or readmission, if discharge instructions are not made clear to the patient or general practitioner (GP). Although the specifics of record keeping or charting may vary according to the type and size of the office or institution and the services offered, it is imperative that good records be maintained in *all* settings. Patient charts are also used as the source of information for billing; funding initiatives; mandatory reporting to governmental bodies; teaching, education, and research; and hospital, regional, and provincial health services planning.

Legal Framework

In order for trust to exist in the physician–patient relationship, patients must be confident that their personal information will be kept strictly confidential. When they are confident, patients are more likely to provide complete and accurate information about their health, allowing the physician to advise and treat them in the way that will be most beneficial.

PRACTICE TIP

When handling information contained in patients' charts, you must always respects their legal rights in accordance with provincial, territorial, and regulatory legislation and guidelines.

Canadian law requires physicians to maintain their patients' health information in confidence. However, each province or territory has specific privacy legislation. Privacy legislation to protect patients' personal health information across the health care system is always developing. The *Personal Health Information Protection Act* (PHIPA) and the *Freedom of Information and Protection of Privacy Act* (FIPPA), together with the College of Physicians and Surgeons of Ontario (CPSO), the Canadian Medical Association (CMA), and the Canadian Medical Protective Association (CMPA), all provide guidelines regarding medical records. These guidelines are intended to ensure the confidentiality and quality of records and to provide the public the right to access their personal information and other government-held data.

Personal Health Information Protection Act (PHIPA)

On November 1, 2004 the ***Personal Health Information Protection Act* (PHIPA)** (pronounced "p-hippa," to distinguish it from FIPPA) became law. PHIPA requires health care personnel to safeguard patients' personal health information against theft, loss, and unauthorized disclosure or use; access only the information they need to do their job; and keep medical records accurate and up to date. Although confidentiality requirements existed prior to PHIPA, the Act has expanded the legal obligations of health care providers in this area.

PHIPA sets out the rules that must be followed when collecting, using, disclosing, securing, transferring, retaining, and destroying a patient's **personal health information (PHI)**, which is defined as identifiable information in oral or written form relating to an individual's health and health care history (for example, OHIP numbers; diagnostic, treatment, and care information; information related to payment; and so on). PHIPA applies to all "health information custodians," including the following:

- all regulated health professionals, including doctors, nurses, dentists, psychologists, optometrists, physiotherapists, chiropractors, massage therapists, social workers, social service workers, and registered dietitians
- non-regulated health professionals who provide health care for payment, such as psychotherapists, naturopaths, nutritionists, and acupuncturists
- the Ministry of Health and Long-Term Care
- Canadian Blood Services
- anyone who operates a hospital; long-term care home; nursing home; psychiatric facility; centre, program, or service for community health or mental health; community care access centre; pharmacy; laboratory; or ambulance service

In addition, PHIPA applies to the agents of information custodians. The Act defines an "agent" as

> a person that, with the authorization of the custodian, acts for or on behalf of the custodian in respect of personal health information for the purposes of the custodian, and not the agent's own purposes, whether or not the agent has the authority to bind the custodian, whether or not the agent is employed by the custodian and whether or not the agent is being remunerated. (s. 2)

As an MA, you are considered an agent and are therefore responsible for ensuring that PHI in the custody or control of the custodian is managed appropriately (s. 17).

DID YOU KNOW?

As an MA, you are an "agent," responsible for ensuring that the requirements outlined in this chapter are met on behalf of the doctor's office, hospital, clinic, or other medical office setting where you will work.

Finally, the Act applies to anyone who receives PHI from a health information custodian. Depending on the situation, this may include an insurance company, employer, researchers, and others.

Physicians must notify any patient whose confidential information has been breached—whether by loss, theft, or unauthorized access—as soon as possible; as an MA, it is your responsibility to notify the physician if you become aware that any of these has occurred. It is an offence to willfully collect, use, or disclose PHI in contravention of PHIPA. The maximum penalty for an individual is $50,000, and for a corporation it increases to $250,000.

PHIPA also affords all individuals the right to access records of their PHI that is in the custody of a health information custodian, subject to certain exceptions.

- The right of access applies to a record, or portion of a record, that is primarily about the individual.

- The right of access does not apply to records that contain quality-of-care information, information required for quality assurance programs, raw data from psychological tests or assessments, or information that is used solely for research purposes and laboratory test results.

- Access to individual records may also be denied if
  - a legal privilege restricting disclosure applies;
  - another law prohibits the disclosure;
  - the information was collected or created for a proceeding;
  - the information was collected or created during an inspection, investigation, or similar procedure;
  - access could result in serious harm to any person, or the identification of a person, who was required to provide information or who has provided the information in confidence; and
  - the custodian is a government institution and the disclosure may be refused under certain provisions contained in access and privacy legislation that applies to government organizations.

Information custodians must respond as soon as possible to written access requests, no later than 30 days after the request and subject to an extension of 30 days. If an individual believes a record is inaccurate or incomplete for the purpose for which it is used, he or she may request in writing that the custodian correct the record. The custodian must correct the record where the individual demonstrates this to be the case, unless one of the exceptions set out in the Act applies.

The following parts of the Act are important for our purposes and will be referred to in this chapter:

- Part I provides *interpretation and application* of the various parts of the Act. It defines and interprets key terms used throughout the legislation. For example, it defines "health custodian" and "agent" as these apply to the Act. It is advisable to read through Part I before tackling the rest of the Act, as it will clarify many of the terms used.

- Part II sets out the *practices* that information custodians must follow to protect PHI—for example, how records should be handled and where they should be kept.

- Part III governs the requirements for the *consent* of an individual or his or her substitute decision-maker before information can be shared or transferred.

- Part IV sets out rules for the *collection, use, and disclosure* of PHI.

- Part V governs individuals' *right to access and correct* their PHI.

Freedom of Information and Protection of Privacy Act (FIPPA)

In 1988, provincial legislation to protect private information called the ***Freedom of Information and Protection of Privacy Act*** **(FIPPA)** came into effect. FIPPA applies to provincial ministries and to most agencies, boards, and commissions in Ontario—for example, local public health agencies or a board of directors for a hospital. It also applies to local health integration networks (LHINs) and hospitals as of January 1, 2012.

Under FIPPA, the government must take certain steps to protect the privacy of personal information contained in government records. Specific rules govern the collection, retention, use, disclosure, and disposal of such information. Under the Act, individuals may also request access to information held by the government, including general records and records that contain their personal information.

FIPPA defines the term "record" broadly. For purposes of the Act, it means

> any record of information however recorded, whether in printed form, on film, by electronic means or otherwise, and includes,
>
> (a) correspondence, a memorandum, a book, a plan, a map, a drawing, a diagram, a pictorial or graphic work, a photograph, a film, a microfilm, a sound recording, a videotape, a machine readable record, any other documentary material, regardless of physical form or characteristics, and any copy thereof. (s. 2(1))

In Ontario, anyone who feels that an institution governed by the Act has compromised his or her privacy can file a complaint with the Information and Privacy Commissioner of Ontario (IPC), who may investigate. Individuals may also request their personal information be corrected if it contains an error or omission.

FIPPA provides the ground rules for determining how federal government departments and agencies handle personal information. The Act provides a right of access to government-controlled information based on the following:

- Information should be available to the public.
- Personal information held by government organizations must be protected, and individuals have a right to access their personal information.

The Act requires that government agencies secure existing records to protect the privacy of an individual's personal information. The Act also recognizes the individual's right to "access government-held information, including general records and records containing their own personal information."[1]

Whether the MA works in a family physician's office, hospital, LHIN, or other medical organization, he or she must always consider the privacy of patients' personal information when writing emails, recording or sharing minutes, transferring medical records, and so on. Under FIPPA, recorded minutes are considered records and are accessible by the public; therefore, when recording meeting minutes, do not include personal information or PHI, such as anything that would help identify the individual—race, nationality, religion, colour, age, sex, marital status, address, or telephone number. If you are working for a hospital or other institution where you are regularly expected to transcribe minutes, review guidelines regarding minute taking, and consider taking additional training in this specialized area.[2]

Protecting Patient Information

To maintain the privacy of patients' personal information, it is important that you follow certain practices and procedures as you work with records and that you store records safely and securely when they are not in use. In this section, we will discuss concerns and proper practices related to technology, phone calls and communication, working with records, and storing records. Although electronic medical records (EMRs) and electronic health records (EHRs) will be referred to in this chapter, they will be explained in greater detail in Chapter 5.

Technology

Despite the many benefits of technology, it brings inherent risks for patient confidentiality. Wireless networks may not be secure; emails may be misdirected accidentally; unauthorized readers may access files; facsimiles may be read by unintended personnel; and special care must be taken to properly erase hard drives on computers and even some photocopiers, and backup copies. Appropriate security measures must always be taken.

Because of the risks involving emails and the fact that they may not be secure, physicians who wish to use this method of transmitting patient information must obtain the patient's express consent to do so (see the discussion of consent, below), unless they have reasonable assurance that the information will be secure when sending and receiving. The College of Physicians and Surgeons of Ontario recommends using a secure email system with strong encryption. The physician may choose a facsimile to transmit patient information. Be aware that anyone who picks up the facsimile will be able to read the information. Always include a cover page stating that the content is confidential using a confidentiality statement (see Appendix 4.1: Fax Cover Page with Confidentiality Statement).

If email correspondence contains PHI, the email author must use a secure server and be confident that the recipient is protecting the PHI. Every organization must have a disclaimer attached to every piece of electronic correspondence, similar to fax correspondence—for example, "This email contains confidential information intended only for the individual or entity named in the message. If the reader of this message is not the intended recipient, or the agent responsible to deliver it to the intended recipient, you are hereby notified that any review, dissemination, distribution or copying of this communication is prohibited."

Phone Calls and Office Communication

All persons discussing patient information—whether over the phone or in person within hearing distance of others—should take precautions to ensure that their conversations are not overheard. This includes MAs.

Ideally, phone calls would be handled in an area where the office administrator would not be overheard. Unfortunately, this is usually not the way offices are set up, and patients in the waiting room may be able to hear you when you are on the phone. It is important, therefore, that you do not reveal too much information about a patient or the patient's chart during the conversation. When leaving a voice message on a machine or with a third party, keep in mind that more than one person may access the messages. Do not include any PHI in your message (e.g., test results, or details about the patient's condition). Leave the name of the physician and contact information, and ask the patient to call back. When playing back your voicemail messages, make sure the volume is not loud enough that patients in the waiting room can hear it. A headset is helpful in this case, as the sound will not be broadcast from a voicemail message.

Whenever possible, keep detailed information in patients' charts about their preferences for being contacted—for example, "okay to leave a message," or "don't leave a message."

A patient's health card information must always be protected. If your computer does not have software that allows you to swipe the patient's health card and you must confirm information orally, be aware of who might overhear. Or ask for the health card and visually confirm the information in the chart with that on the health card. If the patient arrives without his or her health card, the patient must complete a form authorizing you to access the appropriate information from the ministry of health (see Appendix 4.2: Health Card Release Form).

Protecting Charts That Are in Use

While working with patients' charts, you must be careful not to place a chart where anyone may access it or to have it open where a person might be able to see or read it. If you are behind the desk and someone is standing in front of you, be aware that he or she may still be able to read the information, even though the chart is upside down. Always protect a chart that is open on the desk. If another patient arrives while you are consulting a chart, either close the chart or place a blank piece of paper over it to protect the individual's privacy. In the case of electronic files, angle the monitor, minimize the screen, or close the program to ensure that casual onlookers cannot see the PHI displayed. If you must leave your desk, ensure the program is closed and password protected before leaving the computer unattended.

Note that as an office administrator, your contact with charts is limited to when the chart must be pulled for an encounter or updated further to instructions from the physician.

Storing Records

Physicians are ultimately responsible for ensuring that medical records are stored and maintained appropriately. All patient records and data must be kept in locked filing cabinets or otherwise restricted areas to protect against loss of information and damage. Electronic records must be backed up on a routine basis, and back-up copies stored in a physically secure environment separate from where the original data are stored.

The storage location of the medical records—paper or electronic—must be secure. Physicians should be aware of all personnel (including non-medical staff, such as administrative, maintenance, or technical staff) who have access to the records. For electronic records, a password or user identification should be required in order to log on to the system and, where possible, controls should be in place that restrict access based on the user's role and responsibilities. If a physician takes a record out of the office or accesses an electronic record from a location other than her own office, she must handle the record in a way that prevents loss, restricts access, and maintains the privacy of patients' PHI. Appropriate firewalls and virus protection must be installed to protect e-files from external security breaches.

Concern about security for confidential files and documents has existed for a long time. However, with increased technological innovation the concern has grown from keeping hard-copy files and documents secure to keeping documents and files secured when they are stored and shared through mobile devices and cloud computing. It is crucial that an MA be aware of the security risks and has some knowledge of how to secure confidential information.

All confidential or sensitive material should be password protected. Personal computers should have a login password so that unauthorized personnel are unable to access patient files.

PRACTICE TIP

Under PHIPA, agents' actions with respect to patient information are limited to "the purposes of the custodian, and not the agent's own purposes." It is illegal for an MA to just casually retrieve a chart, whether paper or electronic, and read the information in it.

BOX 4.1   Passwords

MS Office provides the following tips for creating a strong password.

A good password…

- Is at least eight characters long.
- Does not contain your user name, real name, or company name.
- Is significantly different from previous passwords.
- Contains characters from each of the following four categories: uppercase letters, lowercase letters, numbers, and symbols.

- When creating the password, avoid complete words. For example, LoveU4Ever* contains all of the tips listed above but contains a full word. It could be changed to Lov3U_4_Ever*.
- Create a password that you will remember without writing it down by relating your password to a favourite sport or hobby. For example, "I love to horseback ride" can be written as a secure password as Iluv#t_hbrid3@.

SOURCE: Adapted from "Tips for Creating a Strong Password," 2014, Microsoft.

All files and documents stored on the computer or on the cloud should also be secure. Word, PDF, Access, and Excel files may be password protected. This will prevent anyone who does access your computer from being able to open confidential documents. In Word, you restrict editing and access to a document through the Developer tab. In Access, Excel, and PDFs, go to the File tab and follow the steps to protect the documents. When creating a PDF file, the software will prompt you to "encrypt file with password." At that point, you will be unable to open the PDF without the password. It is a good idea to destroy the original document.

Universal Serial Bus (USB) keys, public drives, and other storage devices are at risk of compromising confidential information. If you are downloading information to an external storage device, it too must be password protected. Offices often have a shared or public drive where staff can place templates and other items that all staff may need to access. Sometimes files are temporarily downloaded to these drives, potentially allowing access by unauthorized personnel. Consider having this drive password protected as well, allowing only authorized personnel access.

Cloud storage has produced a new set of security concerns. MAs, physicians, and others use cloud for the convenience of accessing files from any location but are unsure of just how secure these documents are. Technology has been developed to alleviate some of this concern, but it still allows access when and where you like. One such development is Transporter, which allows you to share documents, files, media, and other data while keeping it secure.[3]

In some instances—for example, if there is insufficient space in the office—it may be necessary to rely on physical storage of hard-copy files off-site, such as a commercial storage provider, hospital, diagnostic facility, or clinic. In this case, physicians must ensure that authorized parties can still access the medical records when necessary, and that the storage site ensures the physical integrity and confidentiality of the record.

To ensure that all personnel who have access to patient records understand the importance of confidentiality and will uphold it, they are required to sign an Affidavit of Confidentiality. A sample affidavit is included in Appendix 4.3: Confidentiality Agreement.

SCENARIO 4.1

The MA in Dr. Patak's office has been too busy to keep up with the filing, and there is a substantial pile of chart notes not yet filed into individual patient charts. Upon arrival this morning, the MA discovers that the office has been burglarized and along with the theft of the computers, the pile of chart notes has been rifled through.

In the case of the chart notes, has the MA "safeguarded the patients' PHI against theft, loss, and unauthorized disclosure/use," as required by PHIPA? Explain. What about in the case of the computers? Explain.

Collection, Use, and Disclosure of Personal Information

Under PHIPA, the patient's consent is required for the collection, use, and disclosure of PHI, subject to limited exceptions. Consent may be implied or express, and in addition, the requirements of valid consent must be met.

Consent

In the course of providing patient care, physicians routinely share a patient's personal information with others within the patient's health care team. Physicians do *not* need to seek consent from a patient each time they need to do so, but are entitled to assume they have the patient's **implied consent** to share information for the purpose of providing care.

However, PHIPA provides that individuals may expressly instruct that their personal information *not* be collected, used, or disclosed. If the information custodian is aware that a patient has expressly withheld his or her consent, the custodian may not disclose the information. (An exception is made when the custodian believes that disclosure is necessary to reduce or eliminate a significant risk of bodily harm to one or more persons—for example, when a patient threatens to harm himself or others, or in the case of child or spousal abuse.)

In contrast to the implied consent for disclosure related to providing care, in most cases a health information custodian must obtain **express consent** to disclose a patient's personal information to anyone outside the health care team, for example, an insurer or employer, or family members or friends. This is done by having the patient sign a consent form, which is kept in the chart (see Appendix 4.4: Authorization to Release Personal Health Information).

Whether it is implied or express, for consent to be *valid*:

1. It must be the consent of the individual.
2. It must be knowledgeable (that is, the individual must understand the purposes of the collection, use, or disclosure, and must understand that she can give or withhold consent).
3. It must relate to the information.
4. It must not be obtained through deception or coercion.

BOX 4.2   The Physician–Patient Relationship

The physician–patient relationship is one of trust and confidence and is essential when providing health care. The patient must have confidence that the physician will provide high-quality care, and the physician must have confidence that the patient will comply with advice or treatment offered during the course of care. A physician must maintain a professional demeanor, uphold patients' dignity, and respect their privacy.

There are situations in which the physician–patient relationship may be terminated. Because the elements of trust and respect are important, a physician may decide to end the relationship for many reasons. Some examples of when termination of a relationship is recommended include loss of trust through patient fraud (e.g., not disclosing current medications to an emergency room physician in an attempt to acquire more of the drug), physical threat to the physician, or too many missed appointments.

If a physician decides to dismiss a patient from his or her practice, the College of Physicians and Surgeons advises physicians to consider patients' vulnerability and their likely ability to find a new physician in the near future (not always an easy task in Ontario). Physicians may not refuse urgent care until the patient has found a new physician.

A physician may not terminate a physician–patient relationship because the patient is unwilling to pay a block fee or annual fee, or because of race, colour, ethnic origin, sex, gender identity, family status, or any other form of discrimination. The relationship may not be terminated because the patient continually neglects to follow the physician's advice or treatment. The patient has a right to choose whether or not to follow the advice, and the best the physician can do is note the patient's refusal to follow advice in the chart.

To terminate the physician–patient relationship, the physician must notify the patient in writing (see Appendix 4.5: Physician–Patient Relationship Termination Letter). Once the patient has found a new physician, he or she may sign a release form (Appendix 4.4) to have the patient record transferred to the new health care provider.

Capacity and Substitute Decision-Making

PHIPA permits anyone to give or withhold consent to the collection, use, and disclosure of personal information provided he or she has the **capacity** to consent. Capacity means the individual (a) has the ability to understand the information that is relevant to deciding whether to consent to the collection, use, or disclosure; and (b) can appreciate the reasonably foreseeable consequences of giving, not giving, withholding, or withdrawing the consent.

If an individual is under the age of 16, the child's parents are responsible for providing consent. If an individual is deceased, his or her estate trustee must provide consent. Finally, if an information custodian considers an individual *incapable* of providing consent—for example, in the case of a patient with Alzheimer's disease—and the Consent and Capacity Board confirms this determination, consent may be provided by the following substitute decision-makers (in order of rank):

1. the individual's guardian
2. the individual's attorney for personal care
3. the individual's representative appointed by the Consent and Capacity Board
4. the individual's spouse or partner
5. a child or parent of the individual
6. the individual's brother or sister
7. any other relative of the individual

Permitted Collection and Use

The general rule for the collection and use of PHI outlined in PHIPA is that it should be collected directly from individuals and used for the purpose for which it was collected. Most other uses require the patient's express consent. Exceptions to the requirement for consent to use PHI include: for the purpose of obtaining payment for health care; for the planning or delivering of programs or services that the custodian provides or funds; for research purposes (subject to certain conditions); for risk management, for error management, or to improve quality of care; and, as permitted or required by law.

Accessing or using patients' medical records in any manner that is contrary to the legislation may result in significant penalties (see Box 4.3).

BOX 4.3   Improper Use of Records

New Brunswick physician Dr. H. was charged with improperly obtaining medical records on a patient who was no longer under his care. A Board of Inquiry found that in response to a civil suit, Dr. H. had obtained mental health records for a purpose unrelated to the treatment of a patient at the time when the patient was not in his care, and thereby engaged in conduct relevant to the practice of medicine that, having regard to all the circumstances, would be reasonably regarded by Council as disgraceful, dishonourable, or unprofessional.

The Board of Inquiry found the physician guilty of the above charge and made a recommendation on penalty.

At a hearing to consider the penalty, Council heard evidence in support of Dr. H. and ordered the following:

- A suspension of his licence to practise medicine for a period of four months.
- That he submit to an independent psychiatric assessment by an examiner appointed by the College.
- That the completion of such an assessment be a condition of return to practice.
- That he pay the costs of the College. These were subsequently determined to be $29,000.

SOURCE: College of Physicians and Surgeons of New Brunswick. Used with permission.

Releasing Personal Information

As an MA, you will be placed in many situations where disclosure of PHI is requested. The request may come from many sources, including another health care provider, a hospital, a patient's family member, a lawyer, the Ministry of Health and Long-Term Care, or another institution.

Depending on the situation, an individual's PHI may lawfully be disclosed under the following circumstances:

1. based on implied consent
2. based on express consent
3. without the individual's consent (where permitted or required by law)

As noted, patients' PHI is routinely shared with others in the patient's health care team in the course of providing care; express consent is not required in such situations, but rather consent is implied. Understanding when individuals' consent is required to release their PHI is critical because releasing the information without consent in such situations can result in penalties. The physician is ultimately responsible for the transgression, although consequences for physicians vary. Penalties include a reprimand; mandatory continuing education; remedial action to alter practice; and having the medical licence revoked, suspended, or subjected to limitations or modifications. The likely consequence for the MA is dismissal.

In general, express consent is needed when an individual's PHI is disclosed in the following circumstances:

- to someone who is *not* a custodian, and the law does not permit disclosure without consent (e.g., an employer)
- to someone who *is* a custodian but who will not be using the PHI for purposes related to the care of the patient, and the law does not permit disclosure without consent

In most cases, the patient will have signed a consent form instructing which specific bodies/individuals he or she is willing to disclose information to, and in this case, the MA may disclose the information. In a best-practice scenario, the MA should consult with the physician regarding what and how much information to disclose. In cases where information is being disclosed without the patient's consent, it is not up to the MA to decide which information to forward. The physician will make the decision, and the MA will disclose the information on the physician's behalf.

For sample forms authorizing the release of PHI, see Appendix 4.4.

Information about individuals may be disclosed for research purposes and for purposes related to health system planning and management, as long as it is de-identified. To **de-identify** means to remove any information that identifies or could be used to identify the individual (e.g., patient's name, date of birth, OHIP number). The MA will be asked to gather the information and, probably, to remove any identifying demographics.

Lastly, PHIPA includes provisions that permit a custodian, including an MA, as an agent working under the supervision of a custodian (e.g., a primary care physician), to disclose PHI without the consent of the patient in some situations. These include the following:

- where permitted or required by PHIPA or another Act (see Table 4.1)
- in emergencies, where disclosure is necessary for the provision of health care and consent cannot be obtained quickly
- to contact a relative or friend of an injured, incapacitated, or ill client for consent
- to confirm that an individual is a patient or resident in a facility, provide his or her location, and comment on general health status (unless the patient has expressly requested that this information not be shared)

PRACTICE TIP

When you are confronted with a request for PHI, always check the patient's chart for a signed release. If you are unsure what the signed release refers to or how much information you should release, ask the physician or contact the College's Physician Advisory Service, their lawyer, the Canadian Medical Protective Association, or the Information and Privacy Commissioner of Ontario.

TABLE 4.1   Mandatory Disclosure Pursuant to Selected Statutes (no consent required)

Act(s)	Disclosure Made to...	Information Required
Aeronautics Act	Aviation Medical Advisor	Physicians must disclose any information about flight crew members, air traffic controllers, or other aviation licence holders who have a condition that may affect their ability to perform their job safely
Health Protection and Promotion Act and PHIPA	Chief Medical Officer of Health or Medical Officer of Health	Information necessary to diagnose, investigate, prevent, treat, or contain communicable disease
Child and Family Services Act	Children's Aid Society	Information about an abused or neglected child (child in need of protection)
Highway Traffic Act	Registrar of Motor Vehicles	Medical practitioners and optometrists must provide the name, address, and condition of any person who has a condition that may make it unsafe for him or her to drive
PHIPA	Ontario court	Any information sought in a warrant, summons, subpoena, etc.
Vital Statistics Act	Registrar General	Information about births and deaths

SOURCE: Based on data from "Chapter 6 – Disclosure: Giving Personal Health Information to Someone Outside Your Agency," 2014, *Privacy Toolkit*, Canadian Mental Health Association.

- where necessary to eliminate or reduce a significant risk of serious bodily harm to another person or the public
- to the Workplace Safety and Insurance Board, when the Board requires information about an individual who is receiving benefits under the *Workplace Safety and Insurance Act*
- to determine eligibility for government-funded services
- where required by proceedings, including those of a court or tribunal, or a warrant
- where required by an audit or accreditation review
- to designated organizations, in support of health care system management and planning
- for research (as specified in s. 44 of PHIPA)
- to assist in an individual's placement in a facility for health care purposes or in a custodial setting (for example, under the mental disorder provisions in the *Criminal Code*)
- if an individual is deceased, for purposes of identifying him or her and informing persons that the individual is deceased
- to a potential successor, so the successor may assess and evaluate the custodian's practice

Table 4.1 outlines some specific mandatory disclosure requirements under various legislation. Table 4.2 illustrates a number of situations where consent is and is not required, and the authority for releasing the information.

TABLE 4.2 Consent Requirements for Various Types of Disclosure

Requesting Party	Purpose	Consent Required?
Lawyers, insurance companies, or adjusters on behalf of a patient	To assist the patient with a proceeding/claim	Yes (express consent required)
Lawyers, insurance companies, adjusters, or investigators on behalf of a third party (where the third party is or was an agent of the custodian)	To assist the third party with a proceeding	No (PHIPA)
Penal or custodial institution, or a psychiatric facility where a patient is being lawfully detained	To assist with health care or placement decisions	No (PHIPA)
Police with a warrant	For an authorized investigation/inspection	No (PHIPA)
Police without a warrant	Reasonable grounds to believe there is a significant risk of serious bodily harm that can be reduced or eliminated only through disclosure	No (PHIPA) *Note: If the police do not have a warrant and are seeking information for a purpose other than reducing or eliminating a significant risk of serious bodily harm, the best practice is to obtain express consent.*
Probation and Parole Services	Law enforcement	Yes (express consent)

SOURCE: Based on data from "Chapter 6 – Disclosure: Giving Personal Health Information to Someone Outside Your Agency," 2014, *Privacy Toolkit*, Canadian Mental Health Association.

Access to Records

The Supreme Court of Canada ruled in 1992 that the medical record belongs to the physician or health care institution that compiled it. But while the medical chart is the property of the physician, the information contained in the chart is the property of the patient. The patient, therefore, has the right to examine the record and to copy any of the information contained in it, including consultation and other reports obtained from physicians.

The Canadian Medical Association (CMA) holds that physicians should be prepared to provide a copy of the medical record to the patient upon request and to explain the information contained in it. This principle recognizes that patients have control over access to and disclosure of the information compiled about them. If the medical record is to be transferred to another physician for the purposes of patient care, the CMA recommends that the physician who compiled the medical record retain the original documents and forward copies or abstracts (see the following discussion).

SCENARIO 4.2

One of the patients in your physician's practice was in a car accident, and you are aware that he has begun legal proceedings against the other driver. You receive a phone call from the defence lawyer, and she immediately begins to ask you questions about your patient's health condition and the extent of his injuries. She also says that she needs you to forward copies of all of the medical notes that apply to the accident.

Can you provide this information to the lawyer? Why or why not? What should you do?

Transfer of Records

A patient's medical records may be transferred in a number of situations, including at the patient's request; if a physician is relocating and will no longer be seeing a patient; if a physician retires or dies; and if a physician ceases to practise, through not maintaining her certificate of registration.

If the medical record is to be transferred to another physician or facility for the purposes of patient care, the Canadian Medical Association recommends that the physician who compiled the medical record retain the original documents and forward either a copy of the record, a summary, or abstracts. Physicians are required to keep the chart in its entirety for a minimum of ten years in Ontario. Retention periods differ province to province and territory to territory.

The physician must obtain written consent from the patient before proceeding with the transfer. The transfer should be documented in writing, and the documentation should address the location where the original record will be stored for the retention period; the location of the new physician; the transferring physician's right to access the records, if needed, in the future; and the patient's consent to have the records transferred. It is the responsibility of the MA to obtain and retain this information.

The transfer should take place within an appropriate timeframe so that the new physician is able to provide adequate care—as soon as possible, and within 30 days. Transferring records is an uninsured service for which the physician is entitled to charge a reasonable fee, that is, one that reflects the actual cost to the physician in terms of materials, labour, and transfer. The fee may not be requested until after a fee estimate has been given to the patient, but should be paid before the file is transferred, according to the rule set out in PHIPA. A fee may not be requested if withholding the transfer until payment is received would jeopardize the patient's health and safety. Physicians should take the patient's financial circumstances, and his or her ability to pay, into account when considering an appropriate fee.

Retention of Records

In Canada, provincial or territorial legislation, and/or a regulatory authority (e.g., the College that regulates physicians in the particular province or territory), defines the period of time for which a physician must keep clinical records after the date of last entry in the record.

In Ontario, under the *Medicine Act, 1991*, physicians must retain a patient's medical records for 10 years after the last entry date, and hospitals must do so for 10 years after the last visit. For minors, physicians must retain the records until 10 years after the patient reaches or would have reached age 18, and hospitals for 10 years past the age of 18 (age 28).

There are circumstances in which the physician may be required to keep the records for even longer. This is because of a provision in the *Limitations Act, 2002*, which states that some legal proceedings against physicians can be brought 15 years after the act or omission on which the claim is based took place. It is important that the physician be able to provide evidence, should it be required in any future legal proceedings. If a physician's care and treatment of a patient are called into question, the best evidence of treatment is often found in the doctor's notes, which are usually considered a reliable record of the visit. In the absence of any record, the physician will need to defend any allegations from memory, which is likely to have faded with time.

Physicians may also be required to retain records longer than the above time periods when a request for access to personal health information under PHIPA is made before the retention period ends. In such cases, physicians must retain the records for as long as necessary to allow an individual to take any recourse that is available under PHIPA (s. 13(2)). Therefore, regardless of legislation or College policies, the Canadian Medical Protective Association recommends that physicians retain their medical records for at least 15 years from the date of the last entry.

If a physician ceases to practise and is not transferring records to another physician, all patients must be notified that their records will be held for two years. They should also be informed that they may either collect their records or request a transfer to another physician before the end of the two-year period.

If a physician dies or loses his or her licence and can therefore no longer practise, the medical records may be transferred or retained for the same periods outlined by the province or territory. If possible, physicians must make a reasonable effort to give notice to patients of the transfer. If a physician dies before transferring the records, the estate's trustee is responsible for the records until they are transferred to a new physician.

Inactive charts or "dead files"—that is, the charts of patients who have died or whom the physician is no longer seeing—must be stored in a safe and secure location until the retention period is over. A physician's office will usually designate a filing area in the office where these charts are stored, separately from active files. Alternatively, as these files are not needed on hand, they may be stored off-site at a secure location. A record listing dead files, both on- and off-site, should be maintained for ease of retrieval if necessary.

Destruction of Medical Records

A medical record must not be destroyed until the end of the timeframe specified by the province or territory. When the records are destroyed, they must be destroyed in a way that maintains the patient's confidentiality and other requirements of PHIPA. This includes ensuring that the records cannot be reconstructed by anyone at a later date.

The College of Physicians and Surgeons of Ontario requires all paper records to be cross-shredded. The destruction of electronic records is more difficult to accomplish. These must be permanently deleted from all hard drives and any other storage mechanisms. The CPSO requires the drive to be either crushed or wiped clean. These requirements apply to all backup copies as well.

If a patient's records are not destroyed in a manner that protects the patient, the patient could claim breach of confidentiality. The patient may report this breach to the Privacy Commissioner; however, reporting must occur within one year of the incident and be submitted in writing. After investigating the complaint, the Privacy Commissioner may deny the claim or, if the claim is accepted, order the physician to "change, cease or not commence an information practice specified by the Commissioner" (PHIPA, s. 61(1)). Monetary penalties may occur if damages (e.g., mental anguish) are severe enough.

It is important to note that privacy breaches usually occur by accident or negligence on the part of the physician's office, not out of individual malice. As mentioned throughout this chapter, medical offices depend on their MAs to ensure that they are PHIPA-compliant.

The MA must have the physician's approval before destroying a medical record, and the administrator should keep a list of the destroyed records. This will ensure that no questions arise in the future regarding the chart, such as whether it has been lost or misplaced. For each chart that is destroyed, the administrator should include pertinent information on the master list, such as the patient's name and birthdate, date of the last visit, and the date the records were destroyed. Obviously, this list will also require confidentiality protection.

NOTES

1. For more, see "Access to Information Under Ontario's Information and Privacy Acts" at http://www.ipc.on.ca/images/Resources/access-info-e.pdf.

2. Carleton University, for example, offers an excellent source at http://carleton.ca/privacy/wp-content/uploads/minute_taking_tips.pdf.

3. For more information about Transporter, see http://www.filetransporter.com/learn-more/.

RESOURCES

CMPA:
https://www.cmpa-acpm.ca/cmpapd04/docs/ela/goodpracticesguide/pages/communication/Privacy_and_Confidentiality/privacy_and_confidentiality-e.html

Service Ontario, *Personal Health Information Protection Act, 2004*:
http://www.e-laws.gov.on.ca/html/statutes/english/elaws_statutes_04p03_e.htm

REFERENCES

Canadian Mental Health Association (CMHA). (2005). "Chapter 6: Disclosure: Giving personal health information to someone outside your agency." Privacy Toolkit. https://ontario.cmha.ca/public-policy/capacity-building/privacy-toolkit/chapter-6-disclosure-giving-personal-health-information-to-someone-outside-your-agency/.

College of Physicians and Surgeons of Ontario (CPSO). (2000). Policy statement #4-12, 2000, "Medical records."

College of Physicians and Surgeons of Ontario (CPSO). (2006). Policy statement #8-05, "Confidentiality of personal health information." http://www.cpso.on.ca/uploadedFiles/policies/policies/policyitems/Confidentiality.pdf.

Information and Privacy Commissioner. (2004). A guide to the *Personal Health Information Protection Act.* http://www.ipc.on.ca/images/resources/hguide-e.pdf.

Personal Health Information Protection Act, 2004, SO 2004, c. 3, Sched. A.

REVIEW QUESTIONS
True or False?

1. A health record may not be used by the defence in litigation.
2. PHIPA stands for Personal Health Information Privacy Agency.
3. The information in a patient's chart belongs to the physician.
4. Record keeping is a vital component of excellent ongoing health care.
5. Under FIPPA, recorded meeting minutes are considered records and are accessible by the public.

Fill in the Blank

1. Canadian law requires that physicians protect their patients' health information and keep it in _____.
2. An MA is considered by PHIPA to be a(n) _____.
3. Under FIPPA, the government must take certain steps to protect the privacy of personal information contained in _____ records.
4. PHIPA permits anyone to give or withhold consent to the collection, use, and disclosure of personal information provided they have the _____ to consent.
5. Charts of patients who have died or whom the physician is no longer seeing are usually referred to as inactive charts or _____.

Multiple Choice

1. The four main categories of the life cycle of a record are
   a. creation, maintenance, administration, and disposition
   b. creation, maintenance, administration, and transferring
   c. creation, administration, outguiding, and disposition
   d. administration, maintenance, disposition, and delivery

2. For how many years must medical records be retained after the last entry in the record?
   a. 7 years
   b. 5 years
   c. 10 years
   d. 12 years

3. "PHI" stands for
   a. private health information
   b. personal health information
   c. protected health information
   d. privileged health information

4. "Implied consent" refers to
   a. the physician directly asks for your consent to share information
   b. you are required to sign a consent for the physician to share information
   c. the physician assumes you are okay with sharing the information
   d. another person, who is authorized to represent you, gives consent for the physician to share information

5. The patient's chart or health record may NOT be used
   a. as a defence in litigation
   b. as the source information for billing
   c. to post on the Internet
   d. for teaching

6. Which of the following requires consent for disclosure?
   a. police with a warrant
   b. probation officer and parole services
   c. police without a warrant
   d. lawyer acting on behalf of a third party

7. If a patient's records are not destroyed in a manner that protects the patient, the patient can claim breach of confidentiality by reporting the incident to the Privacy Commissioner within
   a. 6 months
   b. 1.5 years
   c. 5 years
   d. 1 year

8. It is important for an MA to understand that a medical record is
   a. something that should be shared
   b. a legal document
   c. a legal document only if the patient is deceased
   d. not a legal document, but should be kept private

9. According to PHIPA, what is the maximum penalty for an individual who breaches the confidentiality of a medical record?
   a. $10,000
   b. $50,000
   c. $250,000
   d. $5 million

Short Answer

1. Explain the difference between implied and express consent. Give an example of each. What three factors demonstrate valid consent?

2. What does "circle of care" mean? What rule applies to the circle of care when dealing with confidentiality?

3. Why is it important for a physician to maintain an accurate patient medical record?

4. In a table, identify methods to protect PHI on a computer and in patient charts (hard copy).

5. Suggest four ways that an MA can ensure the privacy of medical information while at the receptionist window in a medical office.

HYBRID LEARNING

1. Using your school's online discussion board, discuss the following question, and then offer a response to at least one posting. In your own experience when visiting your family doctor's office, what are some of the ways an MA might improve service? In what ways have you witnessed an MA excelling in service?

2. Visit the CMPA website. Under the menu for Education & Events, choose eLearning, and click on Privacy and Confidentiality. Play the video, and then take the challenge quiz to test your knowledge. Submit a screen printout showing completion of the activity (you may skip the Getting Credit section).

ACTIVITIES

1. Read the scenarios below. Using your knowledge of PHIPA, answer the following questions.

SCENARIO 1

A patient requests to view his chart. After receiving permission from the physician, you allow the patient to view his health record. The patient lets the physician know that he would like a correction made to one of the encounter note entries.

a. Does the patient have a right to correct information in the chart?

b. Does the physician have to agree to the correction?

c. What options does the physician have in dealing with changes requested by the patient?

SCENARIO 2

You are the MA at a college health centre. A faculty member calls the health centre asking about the medical condition of a student. The faculty member would also like a medical note to substantiate the student's absence.

a. Can you provide such information about a student's health to a faculty member?

b. Can you provide a medical note? Explain.

c. If the student is okay with PHI being given to the faculty member, what is your responsibility as an MA?

SCENARIO 3

You are working as a unit clerk in the Emergency Room. A man arrives alone, by ambulance with severe facial injuries from a motor vehicle crash. He is unable to communicate. A female calls in distress looking for her husband. She provides enough information to match the information on the man's identification. You believe she is the wife of the man who has arrived with facial injuries. Can you tell her that he is in the ER? Explain.

2. Your physician would like information from a specialist's visit for one of your patients. When you check the chart, you notice that the office has not received a report from the specialist. What are the appropriate steps to take to obtain the information from the specialist?

3. Briefly explain the differences between PHIPA and FIPPA, and their roles with respect to medical records.

4. Find the *Personal Health Information Protection Act, 2004* on the e-Laws website, and review parts I, II, III, and IV of PHIPA. Summarize the information for each part in one paragraph.

5. Re-read Scenario 4.2 on page 79. Choose the appropriate authorization form from the appendices at the end of this chapter, and fill in the patient information. Pay attention to detail. Would you send the form without consulting the physician? Explain.

Patient information: Jeffery Arms, 1015 Abott Street, Kingston, ON K7L 3B5

APPENDIX 4.1

Fax Cover Page with Confidentiality Statement

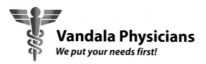

Vandala Physicians
We put your needs first!

400 West Georgia Street
Kingston, ON K6M 3T4
613-224-2308 [telephone]
613-224-2300 [fax]

www.vandala.emp.ca
info@vandala.emp.ca

FAX COVER SHEET

To:

Fax No.:

From:

No. of pages (including cover page):

If pages are missing, please contact:

Comments:

This fax is confidential and is intended only for the person(s) named above. Its contents may also be protected by privilege, and all rights to privilege are expressly claimed and not waived. If you have received this fax in error, please call us immediately and destroy the entire fax. If this fax is not intended for you, any review, distribution, copying, or disclosure of this fax is strictly prohibited.

APPENDIX 4.2

Health Card Release Form

This form is used when a patient arrives for an appointment without his or her health card.

Ontario Ministry of Health and Long-Term Care | Ministère de la Santé et des Soins de longue durée

| Microfilm use only / Réservé aux microfilms |
| Health Number/Numéro de carte Santé | Version |
| Ministry Use Only/Réservé au ministère |

Health Number Release / **Divulgation du numéro de carte Santé**

This form may be submitted to the Ministry of Health and Long-Term Care when the Health Number of a patient is not available.

La présente formule peut être envoyée au ministère de la Santé et des Soins de longue durée lorsque le numéro de carte Santé d'un patient ou d'une patiente n'est pas disponible.

Confidential when completed/Renseignements confidentiels

1. Patient/Patiente

A. General Information/Renseignements généraux

Last name/Nom de famille   First name/Prénom

Middle name/Deuxième prénom   Sex/Sexe   M   F   Birth date/Date de naissance   year/année   month/mois   day/jour

If an alternate last name is known, please provide/Si vous avez un deuxième nom de famille, inscrivez ici

B. Health Number Disclosure/Divulgation du numéro de carte Santé

The Ministry of Health and Long-Term Care will give your Health Number to the health care provider/facility.

I agree to allow the **Ministry of Health and Long-Term Care** to release my **Health Number** to the health care provider/facility listed **below**.

Le ministère de la Santé et des Soins de longue durée donnera votre numéro de carte Santé au fournisseur/à la fournisseuse ou à l'établissement de soins de santé.

J'autorise le ministère de la Santé et des Soins de longue durée à divulguer mon numéro de carte Santé au fournisseur ou à l'établissement de soins de santé dont le nom figure ci-dessous.

Collection of the information on this form is for the assessment and verification of eligibility for Health Insurance and Drug Benefit and administration of the Health Insurance and Ontario Drug Benefit Acts, and for health planning and coordination. It is collected/used for these purposes under the authority of the Ministry of Health Act, section 6(1,2), Health Insurance Act, section 4(2) (b,f), 10, 11(1), and Regulation 201/96 under the Ontario Drug Benefit Act, section 2. For information about collection practices, call 1 800 268–1154, in Toronto (416) 314–5518, or write to the Director, Registration and Claims Branch, P.O. Box 48, 49 Place d'Armes, Kingston ON K7L 5J3.

Les renseignements demandés dans cette formule sont réunis aux fins d'évaluation et de vérification de l'admissibilité à l'assurance-santé et aux prestations de médicaments gratuits, aux fins d'administration de la Loi sur l'assurance-santé et de la Loi de 1986 sur le régime de médicaments gratuits de l'Ontario, et aux fins de planification et de coordination des services de santé. Ces renseignements sont réunis ou utilisés à ces fins en vertu de la Loi sur le ministère de la Santé, paragraphe 6(1),(2), de la Loi sur l'assurance-santé, alinéas 4(2)b),f), article 10, paragraphe 11(1), et du Règlement 201/96 pris en application de la Loi de 1986 sur le régime de médicaments gratuits de l'Ontario, paragraphe 2. Pour plus de précisions sur la collecte de ces renseignements, faites le 1 800 268–1154 ou, à Toronto, le (416) 314–5518, ou écrivez au directeur ou à la directrice de l'inscription et des demandes de règlement, C.P. 48, 49, Place d'Armes, Kingston ON K7L 5J3.

Signature of ☐ applicant ☐ legal guardian ☐ parent ☐ power of attorney   **X**   Date

Home phone number / Téléphone (domicile) (   )   Business phone number / Téléphone (bureau) (   )

A parent or guardian may sign for a child under 16 years of age. An attorney under continuing power of attorney, an attorney under power of personal care, or a legal guardian may also sign on behalf of an individual of any age.

Le père, la mère ou le tuteur, la tutrice peuvent signer pour un enfant de moins de 16 ans.

2. Provider/Facility / Fournisseur/Fournisseuse/Établissement

Provider no./N° du fournisseur   Provider's phone number N° de téléphone du fournisseur (   )   Facility no./N° de l'établissement   Facility phone number N° de téléphone de l'établissement (   ) –

The Health Number of the patient will be returned to the provider/facility listed here.
Le numéro de carte Santé du patient/de la patiente sera transmis au fournisseur/à la fournisseuse/à l'établissement de soins de santé dont le nom figure ci-dessous.

Date of service/Date de prestation du service   year/année   month/mois   day/jour

Provider/Facility name and address/Nom et adresse du fournisseur

Ministry Use Only/Réservé au ministère	
Date received	
Date processed	Processed by

1265–84 (05/03)   ©Queen's Printer for Ontario, 2005   7530–4626

SOURCE: © Queen's Printer for Ontario, 2005. Reproduced with permission. A current version of the form is available on the Government of Ontario's central forms Repository at http://www.forms.ssb.gov.on.ca/mbs/ssb/forms/ssbforms.nsf/FormDetail?openform&ENV=WWE&NO=014-1265-84.

APPENDIX 4.3

Confidentiality Agreement

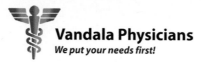

Vandala Physicians
We put your needs first!

400 West Georgia Street
Kingston, ON K6M 3T4
613-224-2308 [telephone]
613-224-2300 [fax]

www.vandala.emp.ca
info@vandala.emp.ca

CONFIDENTIALITY AGREEMENT

I, _____ , an employee of Vandala Physicians (VP), will comply with the *Freedom of Information and Protection of Privacy Act* (FIPPA) privacy module. I understand that I may encounter protected health information during my employment with VP through access and/or availability and that it is my responsibility to maintain confidentiality of this information to the highest standard. I further understand that any breach of confidentiality would result in disciplinary action against me, possible termination of employment, and possible legal action against VP.

_____   _____
Signature   Date

_____
Printed Name

_____   _____
Witness   Date

APPENDIX 4.4

Authorization to Release Personal Health Information

This is a sample form that the patient would be asked to sign authorizing a physician to disclose PHI in order to obtain documents from a hospital or other health care provider.

AUTHORIZATION FOR DISCLOSURE
OF PATIENT INFORMATION

PATIENT

NAME (please include all names if name was different at the time of treatment, i.e., maiden name):

_____

HEALTH CARD NUMBER: _____

DATE OF BIRTH: _____

PHONE: _____

FAX: _____

ADDRESS: _____

AUTHORIZATION

AUTHORIZATION IS HEREBY GRANTED TO: _____

TO RELEASE INFORMATION FROM THE HEALTH RECORD OF THE ABOVE NAMED PATIENT TO:

NAME: _____

PHONE: _____

FAX: _____

ADDRESS: _____

INFORMATION REQUESTED (please specify approximate dates of treatment):

_____

_____

_____

_____

_____

SIGNATURE OF PATIENT OR AUTHORIZED PERSON: _____

This is a sample form that the patient would be asked to sign authorizing a physician or hospital to disclose information to another health care provider or to a court.

CONSENT TO DISCLOSE
PERSONAL HEALTH INFORMATION

Pursuant to the *Personal Health Information Protection Act, 2004* (PHIPA):

I, [print your name] _____ , authorize [print name of health

information custodian] _____ to disclose my personal health

information consisting of [describe the personal health information to be disclosed]: _____

_____

_____

_____

or the personal health information of [name of person for whom you are the substitute decision-maker*]

_____ consisting of [describe the personal health information

to be disclosed] _____

_____

_____

to [print name and address of person requiring the information] _____

_____ .

I understand the purpose for disclosing this personal health information to the person or organization

noted above. I understand that I can refuse to sign this consent form or later withdraw my consent.

My name: _____

Address: _____

Home phone: _____   Work phone: _____

Signature: _____   Date: _____

* Please note: A substitute decision-maker is a person authorized under PHIPA to consent, on behalf of an
   individual, to disclose personal health information about the individual.

APPENDIX 4.5

Physician–Patient Relationship Termination Letter

Dear **[patient's name]**:

As we discussed at your appointment on **[insert date]**,* my first obligation as a medical doctor is to provide quality care to all of my patients. In order to do this, you and I must willingly work together towards your health and well-being.

It has become clear that because of **[if appropriate, indicate reason]**, there has been a breakdown of trust in our doctor–patient relationship. This has made it difficult for me to continue providing quality care to you.

In these circumstances, I do not believe that it is in your best interests for me to continue as your doctor. I, therefore, regret to inform you that I will not be in a position to provide you with further medical services after **[enter the date — this time will vary from community to community, but you should give sufficient notice]**.

I urge you to obtain another physician or primary health care provider as soon as possible. With your consent, I will be pleased to provide them with a copy or summary of your medical records. You can also obtain the results of any outstanding medical tests by contacting **[enter contact information]**.

For assistance in locating another physician, you may wish to call Health Care Connect, a Ministry of Health and Long-Term Care program, which helps Ontarians without a family health care provider find one. To register for the Health Care Connect program, call 1-800-445-1822. Other options include contacting your local hospital to see whether any physicians on staff are accepting new patients, or your Community Health Centre, an organization that provides primary health care and prevention programs through physicians and a variety of other health professionals. A list of community health centres in Ontario is available on the Ontario Ministry of Health and Long-Term Care website. Last, some physicians, including those who are new to an area or who are beginning to establish a practice, will advertise in the local newspaper that they are accepting new patients.

Yours truly,

[signature of physician]

---

* This part may be deleted if the physician has not previously discussed termination of the relationship with the patient.

SOURCE: Used with permission of the College of Physicians and Surgeons of Ontario.

Medical Records 2: Chart Components, Organization, and Filing Systems

5

LEARNING OUTCOMES

After completing this chapter, you should be able to:

- describe the life cycle of a chart
- explain the advantages of electronic records over paper records
- describe the types of records/documents in a physician's office and in a hospital setting, and how to create a medical office patient chart
- identify and describe source- and problem-oriented methods of chart organization
- identify three filing systems, and explain which ones are best suited to particular health care settings
- outline best practices for maintaining the privacy of information contained in patients' charts
- describe different equipment used in filing and understand the importance of file charge-out systems

Failure is simply the opportunity to begin again, this time more intelligently.

—Henry Ford

Introduction

In Chapter 4, we reviewed the legal framework surrounding the personal information that physicians and medical administrators handle on a daily basis, and the general rules governing patient records. (Security and privacy, although the main focus in Chapter 4, will continue to be stressed in this chapter and throughout this book.) Within this context, we will now look more closely at charts themselves—the different formats and components, as well as the systems used in different medical settings to ensure that information in patients' charts is accessible, organized, and secure.

This information is important to a medical office administrator, as you will ultimately be responsible for filing and retrieving charts and overseeing their security, as well as ensuring that the filing system in your health care setting functions effectively and that all charts are accounted for.

Life Cycle of a Chart

Whether a patient is seeking treatment at a doctor's office or a hospital, the patient chart is usually processed according to the following four steps.

1. Creation

When a patient seeks health services, the office administrator in the hospital or medical office records the patient's demographic information and creates labels for the chart. The demographic information in the health record must contain the client's name, address, phone number, birthdate, and health card number. Other important medical and personal information, such as allergies and next of kin, will also be collected. A patient's chart must be accurate, complete, organized, and secure. A new chart cannot be created until the patient requests to join the practice. Creating a chart in the correct way ensures that it can be easily accessed and retrieved whenever needed (see Appendix 5.1: Building the Patient Chart).

2. Maintenance

Patient records within a chart are maintained throughout the life of the patient within the practice (and transferred to the new health care provider if the patient leaves the practice). Each encounter and service rendered must be entered into the chart with the appropriate date. Documentation within the chart is stored in **reverse chronological order**, with the most recent encounter or service appearing first, at the front of the chart. Reverse chronological order is used so that the physician or MA is able to quickly access the most recent and required information. For example, a patient is seen on January 10, and during this encounter the physician orders fasting blood work. Ten days later, on January 20, the patient has another appointment, this time to treat an infected toenail. Then, on January 23, the patient's blood work results arrive. When the MA files the documents, the top document would be the blood work results, the second the infected toenail, and the last one would be the encounter note requesting the fasting blood work.

As discussed in Chapter 4, all patient records and data must be kept in a safe and secure place and protected against loss of information and damage. Charts must also be kept confidential in accordance with provincial/territorial legal guidelines. Electronic health records must be backed up on a daily or nightly basis, and the back-up copies stored in a location other than that where the original data are stored (e.g., on a separate server).

SCENARIO 5.1

A student on a work placement at a medical office is pulling charts when she recognizes the name of a fellow student on a chart. She is curious and reads through the encounter notes. Although she is careful to keep the information to herself, when she returns to the college she attempts to discuss the information with the student.

Has she broken confidentiality? Explain.

3. Administration

Access to and distribution of patient records must be strictly controlled. Charts should never be removed from the premises, and only authorized persons should be allowed access to them. As an MA, you must ensure that patients in the waiting room are not able to view another patient's chart. If you are working with electronic records, always keep the screen turned away or cover the computer screen with a screen protector that prevents easy reading of the screen by other patients or visitors to the office. If you are working with paper records, either close the chart or cover it if a patient approaches the desk. Patients must be notified immediately of any breach of their personal information.

BOX 5.1 Breach of Privacy

Privacy is breached when there is unauthorized access to or disclosure of personal information, including health information. A privacy breach may occur as a result of an administrative error or when personal information is stolen, lost, or mistakenly disclosed (e.g., computer virus, theft, or mailed through Canada Post or email to the incorrect individual).

The Office of the Privacy Commissioner of Canada (OPC) is responsible for investigating cases in which privacy is breached. Its first step is to open an incident file, but an in-depth investigation does not occur unless no steps are being taken to address the situation or to prevent a recurrence.

The OPC recommends the following steps for responding to a privacy breach:

1. Immediately stop the breach—revoke computer access codes, and shut down the system.

2. Evaluate the risks associated with the breach—before you act, determine what information was breached and the sensitivity of the information. This will help you determine who, if anyone, should be informed of the breach.

3. If a privacy breach creates a risk of harm to the individual(s), those affected should be notified. Notify the individual(s) as soon as possible by letter, phone, or email, or in person. (If the breach involves law enforcement, check before notifying individuals of breach.)

SOURCE: Based on "Guidelines: Key Steps for Organizations in Responding to Privacy Breaches," 2007, Office of the Privacy Commissioner of Canada.

4. Disposition

Where and how a record is stored or archived, and when it may be destroyed, varies depending on the situation. Refer to the guidelines in Chapter 4.

Electronic Records

Electronic health information is grouped into three categories: the **electronic medical record (EMR)**, the **electronic health record (EHR)**, and the **personal health record (PHR)**. These categories are computer-based medical information systems. The terms EMR and EHR are often used interchangeably, but they refer to different things:

- An EMR is a patient record maintained by a physician over time—essentially, a chart, but in electronic form.

- An EHR is a compilation of a patient's health data from multiple sources, made up of records submitted by numerous providers and organizations (e.g., specialists, hospitals, nursing homes) and accessible to everyone in the patient's health care team.

- A PHR is another form of electronic medical record. It is used by the patient to keep track of past and future medical appointments, lists of medications and treatments, correspondence (whether electronic or hard-copy) with health care providers, and an immunization schedule. A PHR may take the form of emails, electronic calendars for tracking appointments, and chat rooms for sharing medical information.

> **DID YOU KNOW?**
>
> Since 2001, Canada has been trying to implement EHRs to provide a better and more efficient health care system. However, the country has been slow to adopt this method of charting. In 2007, only 23 percent of Canadian physicians were using EHRs. By 2013, 57 percent of primary care physicians were using EHRs.

Electronic records facilitate the delivery of more efficient care. Without them, patients' health records—diagnostic test results, blood tests, paperwork from a walk-in clinic, prescriptions, and so on—may exist in any number of locations across the country and would not be in a single centralized location. Diagnosis and treatment may be delayed or hampered by missing and incomplete information. With electronic records, however, all such critical information can, in theory, be housed securely online and accessed by anyone who requires it and is authorized to obtain it. EMRs offer many benefits to both physicians and patients, and current technological advances demonstrate future potential. For example, the technology enables alerts to help physicians keep track of immunization schedules and allergies, and prompts for patient follow-up, diagnostic testing, or prescription renewal.

Electronic records replace paper charts and allow lab reports, diagnostic test results, insurance information, and other records to be easily and quickly integrated into the patient's chart. As soon as the patient information has been inputted into the EHR, it is accessible by all health care providers dealing with shared patients and permits faster access to test results and more accurate patient records. Each health care provider adds to the patient's chart, eventually building an EHR that provides an important link among all those involved in the patient's care and treatment. Once EHRs are implemented more broadly, it is anticipated that their use will reduce wait times, provide more efficient management of chronic diseases, and improve access to care in remote and rural communities.

Electronic records offer access to patient information by any networked computer in the office; some facilities (but not many yet) also allow networking between institutions. For example, a family physician's office may be linked to an imaging office, and after a patient has an imaging test, the results will be downloaded directly to that patient's file in the medical office. Currently, most electronic files or images are sent via email, and the MA downloads the results to the patient's EHR. There is no doubt that EHRs are improving the efficiency, safety, and team approach of health care.

Physicians are able to complete a variety of tasks simultaneously using electronic records, including reviewing lab reports and patient history, ordering tests, and prescribing medications. EMRs also allow for easy reporting of and access to research data, practice demographics and statistics, and any other information the physician may want to compile for research, funding, or practice analysis. For example, if a physician requires a report on all female patients between the ages of 20 and 40 who have a regular Pap test, the office administrator can set those parameters within the EMR and generate a report. Without an EMR, the MA would have to search each chart manually, and then amalgamate the information for the report. EMR searches can also help ensure that patients are tested according to the billing guidelines, and not more frequently than is permitted. For example, in Ontario, a patient whose Pap results are normal may be tested only once every three years; if the test is done more frequently, the physician is not permitted to bill for the testing.

The development of EMRs and EHRs, while improving health care, has also provided some challenges: controlling access to patients' personal information, preventing destruction or loss of electronic files, and ensuring the privacy and security of patient records. Ensuring that chart information is accessible only by password, limiting the number of people with access, adding firewalls, and using a server to back up data all assist in protecting patient charts from loss, corruption, or misuse.

EMRs and EHRs are expensive, and the cost to purchase, maintain, and train staff on the software deter some physicians from investing. Standard requirements for EMR software do not exist, and this factor also may make accessing files from other health care organizations, pharmacies, and others difficult.

The rules described for paper filing apply to electronic filing as well. However, additional rules are being developed to accommodate differences in managing, storing, accessing, and destroying EMRs. The Canadian Medical Protective Association (CMPA) has identified the following areas where rules are still being evaluated and adapted:

- ownership of data
- privacy and consent
- access to and accuracy of information
- evidentiary requirements (e.g., a patient's health record may be used in court if quality of care is questioned)

Many physicians are still transitioning from paper to electronic records. Items that must be converted to electronic form include requisitions, reports, progress notes, and handwritten comments. This process is time consuming because ensuring that each patient's information is correctly entered into the computer involves many hours of data entry and scanning of documents. There is always a potential for human error while entering data into the computer chart, and it is essential that the MA keep track of all scanned material so that, once it has been copied to the chart, all other saved copies are destroyed and not left accessible on the computer's hard drive. Both the MA and the physician must be careful to protect patients' personal health information (PHI) while the transition takes place, though it is the physician who ultimately bears the responsibility for maintaining the integrity and privacy of patients' information.

PRACTICE TIP

The same rules apply to the management of both paper and electronic records. However, as rules for electronic records are still emerging, it is important to remain aware of developments in this area.

Many physicians maintain both a paper chart and an electronic chart for each of their patients. Physicians who are converting paper charts to electronic records and who plan to use only electronic charts going forward may destroy the paper chart *only* if the following conditions are met:

- written procedures for scanning are developed and followed
- safeguards to ensure the reliability of digital copies are in place
- a quality assurance process is established, followed, and documented (e.g., comparing scanned copies to originals to ensure accuracy)
- the scanned copies are saved in "read-only" format

If files are converted to searchable and editable files using optical character recognition (OCR) technology, the original record or a scanned copy must be retained. Records that have been converted using voice recognition software must also be retained according to the retention periods set out in Chapter 4.

BOX 5.2 The Right to Privacy Up in Smoke

In 2013, Health Canada sent out letters to recipients of medicinal marijuana, explaining changes being made to the medical marijuana program. Unfortunately, these particular letters were mailed in envelopes that clearly stated who the correspondence was coming from—Marijuana Medical Access Program, Health Canada—thereby breaching the patients' privacy.

According to Health Canada, approximately 40,000 letters were mailed, and the labelling was an administrative error. Health Canada regrets the error and is taking steps to prevent it from happening again.

A law firm has filed a class-action lawsuit against the federal government over the privacy breach. If the suit is successful, all 40,000 Canadians who received the envelopes would benefit.

SOURCE: Based on "Medical Marijuana User Accuses Health Canada of Privacy Breach," November 22, 2013, CBC News.

Components of a Chart

Patient charts contain a range of information, including progress notes; reports; family history; physicians' opinions on patients' condition and care; and information on past and present illnesses, treatments, and tests. A patient's medical health record in a doctor's office may include the following documentation (the information would also be found in a hospital record, but the setup differs):

- *Patient profile (PP).* Also known as the cumulative patient profile (CPP), this must be maintained for each patient. The PP contains a brief summary of essential information about the patient, including:
  - patient identification (name, address, phone number, health card number)
  - history/interview sheet (contains demographics)
  - family history
  - past medical history
  - risk factors

- ongoing health concerns
- allergies and drug reactions

The PP provides anyone who views the chart with a more complete understanding of the patient's overall health.

- *Problem list.* This is located on the inside cover of the chart and in the patient profile, for electronic charts. It lists current medications, long-term problems, and allergies. The location of this document permits easy referral when looking at ongoing health concerns and medications.

- *Progress notes.* These are the clinical notes that are dictated or recorded at each patient visit.

- *Physical assessments.* Any assessments, such as a Pap or annual physical, are recorded on a separate document or may be attached to the PP.

- *Laboratory results reports.* Documents received from diagnostic laboratories or imaging departments are placed at the front of the chart in reverse chronological order for easy access, and not necessarily with the encounter note in which the test was requested.

- *Consent forms.* These are the documents that have authorized the physician to share medical record information with the person(s) specified in the document. (See the discussion on consent in Chapter 4.)

Chart Organization

There are different ways to approach the organization of charts, each with its advantages and disadvantages. This text will focus on two: source-oriented medical records and problem-oriented medical records.

Appendix 5.1: Building the Patient Chart contains instructions for creating a patient chart.

Source-Oriented Medical Records

In **source-oriented medical records (SOMRs)**, charts are organized into sections. Each section is based on the type of medical information in the report or where the report originated. The record is divided by subject matter or source of origin (e.g., lab reports are all kept together, as are progress reports), and each subject or source has a tab or an index in the chart (see Figure 5.8).

SOMRs make it easy to locate some documents quickly, but difficult for the physician to collect all of the various documents in support of a diagnosis. For example, because all diagnostic reports are filed under the "Diagnostic Reports" tab and all progress reports are filed under the "Progress Reports" tab, if a physician requests all of the documentation regarding the condition of a patient's knee, the MA is easily able to retrieve the diagnostic report labelled "knee X-ray," but then must go to the progress section to retrieve the physician's notes, and may also have to find results under the "Laboratory Reports" tab and the "Medications" tab to assemble all the relevant documentation for the physician.

While the retrieval of this type of documentation is often simplified in EHRs, the MA must still open several windows to retrieve all documentation from the patient's chart. Working with several windows may increase the risk of the MA's missing pertinent information. If the MA is unaware of a test requisition, for example, it may not be retrieved and brought to the physician's attention.

> **PRACTICE TIP**
>
> If you are managing paper charts, if any received test results are printed on paper smaller than an 8.5 x 11-inch sheet, staple the results to a blank 8.5 x 11-inch sheet so that they are not lost or misplaced inside the chart.

Problem-Oriented Medical Records

The **problem-oriented medical record (POMR)** method arranges the chart in reverse chronological order according to the patient's most recent complaint or last visit. It treats each patient visit as a complaint that will require further action. The action is determined using the following four categories:

- *Database.* The database provides the physician with the information needed to diagnose a problem. It includes the primary care provider's patient history, social and family data, and the results of the physical examination and baseline diagnostic tests.
- *Problem list.* All of the patient's problems are compiled into a list that is kept at the front of the chart.
- *Plan.* The physician takes all the information gathered above (in the database and the problem list) and develops a plan. The plan may be therapeutic or diagnostic, or involve patient education. For example, the plan for a patient who has been diagnosed with diabetes might contain a therapeutic element (medication) and an educational element (dietary training).
- *Progress notes.* These are the notes that the physician enters into the patient's chart at each encounter. They contain a summary of the discussion during the encounter, any medication prescribed, whether a consult was requested, and any follow-up information.

POMRs allow physicians and other health care providers to easily follow a patient's course of treatment and progress for a particular problem; however, this method makes it more difficult to determine whether past treatments or results have any bearing on the current problem. For example, a patient is seen complaining of fatigue, feeling cold, and having difficulty concentrating. Suspecting low iron, the physician orders the appropriate blood work. At the follow-up visit, the blood work shows very low iron and hemoglobin counts. The physician flips through the chart looking for previous blood work results before deciding on a course of treatment, but may be unable to locate the last blood work results.

Hospital Records

The components of a hospital record differ somewhat from those of a general practitioner's chart. Each patient who is admitted has a record of care, and many departments within the hospital contribute to the care of patients.

Like an office chart, a hospital chart provides the basis for patient care, serves as a legal record, and may be used as a data source for research. Unlike many doctor's office charts, a hospital chart always has an electronic component and a paper component. The paper component is usually housed in a small binder rather than a manila file folder. The binder is usually located at the nurses' station on each ward and is accessed by the nurses, unit clerks, physicians, and other health care providers. It contains progress and daily activities, and is usually divided into the following six sections:

- *Medical documentation.* This section contains the patient's medical history, consultations, physicians' orders, anesthetic record, treatment records, and progress notes.
- *Nursing documentation.* This section contains the patient profile, assessment database, comprehensive patient care record, progress notes, vital signs record, activity of daily living sheets, continuous parenteral therapy record, fluid balance record, and the medical administration record (MAR).
- *Laboratory data.* This section is usually found at the front of the chart, often in a plastic sleeve. It contains the lab results of any tests that are performed.

- *Admission detail.* This is a sheet from Patient Admissions detailing the patient's demographics and next of kin, usually located at the back of the chart.
- *Discharge plan.* This section covers the discharge instructions and any other information the patient should know when leaving the hospital (e.g., prescriptions and home care). The patient is provided with a copy.
- *Discharge sheet.* This sheet provides the details of the patient's admission, treatment(s), procedure(s), discharge medications, follow-up, any further instructions, and a discharge date. It is completed by the physician.

The Patient Records department is responsible for all of the patient charts in a hospital. After a patient is discharged, the patient's chart is kept on the hospital floor for two days and is then sent to the Patient Records department. The chart can be accessed, if necessary, at a later date.

The exact setup of a hospital chart will be looked at in detail in Chapter 10.

Filing Systems

Filing is the process of organizing health records on a shelf, in a filing cabinet, or in an electronic database. Both types of file storage must consider space, efficiency, organization, and security.

Before an MA can create or file a chart, whether in paper or in electronic form, he or she must have knowledge of the different types of filing systems available and the one that is in use in the particular office environment. Whether charts are filed electronically or manually, the office must decide on a method. Types of filing and Association of Records Managers and Administrators (ARMA) filing rules are only briefly reviewed in the sections below; a detailed explanation appears in Appendix 5.2: ARMA Filing Rules.

BOX 5.3	Association of Records Managers and Administrators

The Association of Records Managers and Administrators (ARMA) is a not-for-profit professional association established in 1955. It is the leading association providing education and resources for records and information management and is the author of the filing rules used today. ARMA Canada has 14 chapters across Canada and approximately 1,800 members. Members include information managers, archivists, corporate librarians, imaging specialists, legal and health care professionals, educators, and IT managers.

SOURCE: Based on information from ARMA International.

Dealing with and filing various incoming and outgoing documents is a large part of the MA's daily routine, and it is important for the MA to be familiar with the terms *annotating, cross-referencing, indexing,* and *coding.*

An MA will often be responsible for **annotating** correspondence and for interpreting the annotations that physicians use in patient charts. Annotating is a method of summarizing or highlighting the key information in a document. For example, if a physician receives a letter asking him to attend a medical conference, the MA may annotate the letter by highlighting the date of the conference, important information, and the need for an action/response on the part of the physician. Figure 5.1 shows an example of annotation by an MA.

The MA will also need to interpret physician annotations. Figures 5.2 and 5.3 are examples of physicians' annotations on laboratory reports.

Cross-referencing is another important tool for managing charts and documentation. A cross-reference allows the MA to connect one chart to another chart, such as in the case of

FIGURE 5.1   Annotation: Conference Invitation

January 8, 2014

Rec'd Jan 10/14

av

Vandala Physicians
400 West Georgia Street
Kingson, ON   K6M 3T4

Dear Physicians,

ENDOCRINOLOGY PRIMARY CARE CONFERENCE

We would like to invite you to our Endocrinology Primary Care Conference from April 14, 2014 to April 17, 2014. Our conference will help physicians accurately recognize presenting signs and symptoms of commonly seen disorders; identify available tests for diagnosis, and their appropriate application in making a diagnosis; and apply available treatment options and relevant long-term care, as may be indicated.

The cost per physician for the Conference is $1,625.00. This includes accommodation, meals, and conference sessions. Registration deadline is April 1, 2014.

Please see the attached brochure for more detailed information and a registration form.

We look forward to hearing from you soon.

Sincerely,

MEDICAL TECHNOLOGIES

Pat Lydell

Pat Lydell
Executive Director

*Please let me know
if you would like
to attend*

av

PL/av

FIGURE 5.2   Lab Report Annotation 1

```
2015/02/14  17:01:54                                      P. 001/001

                                    CUSTOMER SERVICE PHONE/FAX REPORT
---------------------------------------------------------------------
OMNICARE LABS               COLLECTION TIME    AEA 50-14020326   REPRINT
123 CHRIS HADFIELD BLVD.     2015/01/18
BURLINGTON, ON L7T 3M5
                                                          2015/02/14

Patient Demographics        0000000001                   Dr. Vandala
                                                     Vandala Physicians

PHONE: 416-555-0000         F     35 Y         PHONE: 613-555-0000

                                                                AEA
                                                          6     A
                                                        271     F
                                                        615     W

* * * * * * * * * * * * * * * * * * * * * * * * * * * * * * * * * * * * * *
This report is intended only for the use of the addressee and contains
confidential information. Any dissemination of this information is prohibited.
If you have received this report in error, please notify the sender.
* * * * * * * * * * * * * * * * * * * * * * * * * * * * * * * * * * * * * *

                          C H E M I S T R Y
                          ------------------
```

CODE	TEST	DESCRIPTION	RESULTS	REFERENCE RANGE	OUTSIDE NORMAL LIMITS
	sTSK		3.84	0.35 – 5.00 mu/L	
R	T4 FREE		6.	10 – 20 pmol/L	6.
	FREE T3		3.0	2.6 – 5.7 pmol/L	
	CORTISOL	RANDOM	977.	65 – 540 pmol/L	977.

Book f/u with patient 3/52

mv

```
              PAGE 1 OF 1  2015/02/14  17:00:25
```

FIGURE 5.3   Lab Report Annotation 2

LifeLabs
Medical Laboratory Services   Inquiries: (877) 849-3637

CYTOLOGY NUMBER
GY-13-TO-000006

DATE OF BIRTH	PATIENT SURNAME	

CLIENT   Route: 7200   Stop: 9313

DR. Sheila BOSS
Dr. Sheila Boss
100 International Blvd
Toronto , ON M9W 6J6

SEX	AGE	FIRST NAME
F		

CHART

HEALTH NUMBER   TELEPHONE NUMBER
( )   -

LIFELABS NO
170230062013

SERVICE DATE   REPORT DATE

CYTOPATHOLOGY REPORT

TYPE OF SPECIMEN: PAP / Liquid Based

SPECIMEN ADEQUACY: Satisfactory for evaluation :
Transformation zone components identified.

INTERPRETATION: **NEGATIVE FOR INTRAEPITHELIAL LESION OR MALIGNANCY :**
BENIGN ENDOCERVICAL COLUMNAR CELLS IN A WOMAN WITH A
PREVIOUS HYSTERECTOMY.

RECOMMENDATIONS: Benign endocervical columnar cells in a Pap from a woman with a previous
hysterectomy may be due to residual cervical tissue, vaginal adenosis or other
benign conditions. This finding in itself is not normally considered an indication
for further action.

CLINICAL HISTORY   Date Taken: 2013 01 15
Post Partum (Wk):   Test
Post Menopause: Test

NOTE:
Pap tests help screen for cervical cancer and its precursors, both false positive and false negative results may occur. The test should be
used at regular intervals, and positive results should be confirmed before definitive therapy. Any visible cervical abnormalities and/ or
abnormal symptoms must be investigated regardless of cytologic findings.
If the Pap test is "Negative for Intraepithelial Lesion or Malignancy" and there is no recent history of abnormal results, significant
immunosuppression or other indication, screening should be done every 3 years after the age of 21. Screening may be discontinued at the
age of 70 if there is an adequate negative cytology screening history in the previous 10 years.
References for more detail:
Ontario Cervical Screening Cytology Guidelines, May, 2012 www.cancercare.on.ca/screenforlife.

Refer to gynecologist
for review of test
mv

Cytotechnologist: 1NB

Pathologist:
Dr. Kim It TEST M.D., Pathologist

100 International Blvd., Toronto M9W 6J6

Page 1 of 1

a patient who marries or divorces and therefore has a name change. Another common use for a cross-reference is when it is difficult to determine which part of a name is the first and which the last—for example, Henry James or James Henry.

Indexing is the most important part of any filing system. The most popular and effective indexing systems are described below.

Alphabetical Filing

In alphabetical filing, medical records or charts are organized by patient surname, from A to Z. The other two main types of alphabetical filing are *subject filing* and *geographic filing* (both described below).

The alphabetical filing method is the most common filing method in medical offices. It is easy to manage and understand, and requires no separate index for identification (i.e., to link a patient to his or her corresponding chart). However, it does not offer any confidentiality; patients can easily be identified by their surnames. Subject filing and geographic filing offer better confidentiality and also ease of locating related information.

Subject Filing

As the name implies, **subject filing** stores and retrieves documents alphabetically according to their subject. It is a convenient system to use when the purpose is to keep all records on a certain topic together. A physician who is studying ovarian cancer, for example, might set up subject filing as follows:

> *Primary Guide:* "O"
> *Secondary Guide:* Ovarian Cancer (documents behind the guide may be organized further by age, weight, or other characteristics)

Filing by subject is also commonly used for "in-office" filing, such as rent, utilities, equipment, and supplies. Documents filed by subject are usually coded. **Coding** is the physical act of marking the filing units or system on correspondence to be filed. For example, information received from Abbott Diabetes Care regarding faulty test strips could be filed under several subjects—diabetes, recalls, pharmaceutical companies—so it must be coded for proper filing. The MA would underline or write the code word on the document to demonstrate where the letter should be filed, in this case, Recalls (Figure 5.4).

Geographic Filing

Geographic filing organizes records according to geographic location or area—towns, counties, neighbourhoods, and so on. This type of filing is often used by real estate agents, catalogue distributors, political organizations, and other agencies. It is not usually used in medical offices or hospitals.

Numeric Filing

Numeric filing is a useful method for indexing large systems, as several digits can be colour-coded and there is little confusion as to where a number falls in a sequence. Straight numeric filing requires an index or cross-reference file to link the patient to his or her number, and is therefore somewhat more complicated—though it does have the benefit of offering confidentiality. This type of filing is rarely used in medical office settings but is common in hospitals and larger organizations.

FIGURE 5.4   Recall Letter

ONTARIO DIABETES SOLUTION
SUPERCARE
BLOOD GLUCOSE TEST STRIPS

ERRONEOUSLY LOW BLOOD GLUCOSE RESULTS

USE: Supercare Blood Glucose Test Strips are used by health care professionals and people with diabetes to monitor blood glucose levels. Blood glucose test strips measure the amount of glucose (sugar) in a blood sample collected by pricking the skin.

RECALLING FIRM: Ontario Diabetes Solution
15 Bloor St. West
Toronto, ON M5A 1J6

REASON FOR RECALL: Affected Supercare Blood Glucose Test Strips may deliver erroneously low blood glucose results. An erroneously low blood glucose result may lead to failure to diagnose and appropriately treat high blood sugar (hyperglycemia) or inappropriate treatment. Treatment of an erroneously low glucose result may lead to too much carbohydrate intake or insulin under dose, and could result in hyperglycemia and other serious adverse health consequences, including death.

PUBLIC CONTACT: For questions about this recall, contact Ontario Diabetes Solution Customer Service at **1-800-555-1212**.

There are several types of numeric filing: *consecutive numbering* (also called *serial numbering, sequential numbering, straight numbering*), *terminal digit filing*, and *chronological filing*. Consecutive numbering involves numbers that are in correct counting order. For example, 1, 2, 3, or 25, 26, 27, 28.

Terminal digit filing is used when there is a very large number of files. Hospitals and other institutions use this system most often. The numbers may be divided into pairs or groupings of three. The complexity of this filing system ensures patient confidentiality and allows files to be numbered in advance. For example, the file number "12-23-54" would mean that the document is number 54 and is filed in drawer 12, behind section 23.

In chronological filing, files are ordered according to dates—most commonly, reverse chronological filing is used, with the file that was used most recently placed on the top, or alternatively, the item within a file that was used most recently placed first within the file. This type of filing system is rarely used to arrange charts in a medical office; however, it is the most common method for organizing the *inside* of each patient's chart, as explained earlier in regard to problem-oriented medical records.

Alphanumeric Filing

Alphanumeric filing combines letters and numbers to identify folder contents accurately. It is often used in hospitals and large institutions. This system offers confidentiality but may be more difficult to grasp than straight alphabetical or numerical systems.

The letters in an alphanumeric system correspond to the patient's last name, and the numbers may denote either the patient's number in the order of arrival of patients or the date of the patient's first visit. For example, John Smith arrives for his first appointment and is the 3,014th patient on record at the hospital. His chart would be labelled "3014Smith."

In both alphabetical and numeric filing, the charts are identified by coloured tabs. Each letter or number is colour-coded (see Figure 5.8).

Manual (Paper Record) Storage

Storing records in paper form requires a considerable amount of equipment. Beyond the forms that organize medical information, a sophisticated filing system is needed to ensure that files are not mixed up or lost.

Medical offices use specific equipment to keep patient records organized and secure, and it is sometimes the responsibility of the MA to select and order this equipment. If the responsibility of choosing equipment falls to you, keep in mind that filing cabinets or storage units are bulky, and consider such factors as floor space, accessibility, security (in terms of the room and the cabinet itself), and appearance.

To ensure confidentiality, access to patient charts should at all times be restricted to medical office administrators, physicians, and other health care personnel (including outside of office hours).

Open-Shelf Filing

The best manual filing setup for charts is open-shelf filing using a lateral filing cabinet or "bay" type of shelf. Lateral filing cabinets are upright shelving units that resemble a bookcase with panel doors (Figure 5.5).

Typically, the panel doors slide upward, like a garage door, and are tucked in above the charts. Lateral or open-shelf files are popular in medical offices because, unlike the vertical filing cabinets described below, they don't open by extending a drawer. This makes them

FIGURE 5.5   Open-Shelf Filing

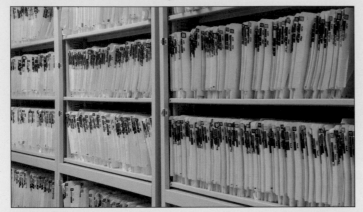

SOURCE: Inka One/iStock/Thinkstock.

FIGURE 5.6   High-Density Storage Units

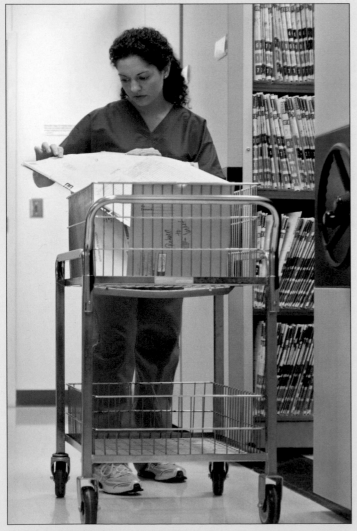

SOURCE: Fuse/Thinkstock.

more compact than vertical filing cabinets. As well, because lateral filing cabinets are usually left open during office hours, accessing files is easy. The shelves have vertical supports, so charts are stored in an upright position with the tabs and colour-coded labels extending out. The fact that the labels are clearly visible helps prevent misfiling and permits easy locating of charts.

Although we have identified this type of filing as open-shelf filing, it differs slightly from true open-shelf filing, in which the cabinet does not have a back or doors that can be secured to protect the contents. True open-shelf cabinets do not maintain privacy and may also be less sturdy than other types of filing cabinets, as they have only end supports. For this reason, they are not suitable for medical office environments.

Lateral filing cabinets may also be purchased with rolling units (Figure 5.6). These high-density storage units convert traditional vertical filing cabinets into one, two, or more movable cabinets. This allows the office to condense filing and free valuable floor space.

Vertical Filing Cabinets

Not all files in a medical office are patient records, and other files must be stored separately from patient charts. These "in-office" files may include such items as employee records, payroll, insurance, supply lists, rent, accounts payable, and hydro.

The traditional vertical, or upright, filing cabinet with three to five drawers is still used in medical offices to store other business records. These cabinets tip easily and must have a safety feature in place: either a wall anchor or a fail-safe mechanism that allows only one drawer to open at a time. Vertical filing cabinets take up more space when a drawer is pulled out. An open drawer may block traffic flow or cause injury, so thoughtful placement is important.

PRACTICE TIP

It is a good idea not to file charts on the bottom shelf, as they are more at risk of being damaged, and storing and retrieval may be difficult. As a safety precaution, charts should not be filed on the top shelf if it means the office administrator will require a stepping stool to access them.

File Folders

Medical file folders (Figure 5.7) have a longer back page, which provides a tab on which to place colour-coded labels. Information may be placed both inside and outside the folder. Information on the outside of the chart might include basic but important information, such as the patient's name, birthdate, allergies, and drug reactions. More detailed patient information, including SOAP notes, medications, referrals, test results, and so on, are placed in reverse chronological order on the inside of the folder. **SOAP** notes are chart notes that follow a specific format—*Subjective*, *Objective*, *Assessment*, and *Plan*. The physician dictates information for each or some of the headings in his or her chart note.

All of the manual filing methods described in this chapter may use colour-coded end filing tab folders (Figure 5.8). Colour-coded end filing is used by the majority of all paper-filing medical institutions. Coloured alpha and numeric characters are available from medical filing suppliers.

Each letter and number has a distinct colour. When the coloured characters are placed on the folder tabs and the folders are filed on the shelf in order, it is easy to identify any charts that have been misfiled (Figure 5.9).

PRACTICE TIP

Practise a few simple rules to lighten the burden of filing:

- Leave space in each alphabetic section for new charts and so that you can easily retrieve and replace charts.
- Never pull out the chart using the tab; this will preserve the file longer and avoid tearing off the tab.
- Always return the chart to the correct file location and in the correct position (i.e., right side up and facing in same direction).
- Whenever possible, file charts immediately so that charts to be filed do not pile up.
- Create a very specific area in the offices where files are placed (e.g., in and out boxes).
- To avoid misplacing test results or other documentation, replace any papers removed from the chart as soon as possible.

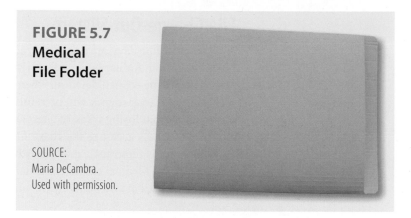

FIGURE 5.7
Medical File Folder

SOURCE:
Maria DeCambra.
Used with permission.

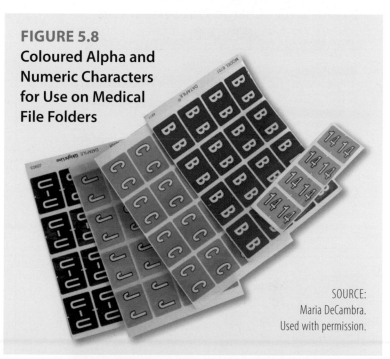

FIGURE 5.8
Coloured Alpha and Numeric Characters for Use on Medical File Folders

SOURCE:
Maria DeCambra.
Used with permission.

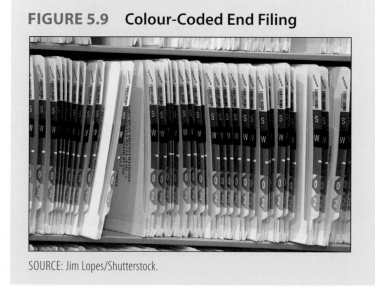

FIGURE 5.9   Colour-Coded End Filing

SOURCE: Jim Lopes/Shutterstock.

File Charge-Out System

A system must be developed to keep track of charts when they have been removed for purposes other than for use while the patient is in the office or hospital. When this happens, a record should be created detailing when the file was removed, who has the file, why the file was removed, and when it will be returned. A **charge-out system** prevents the office administrator from losing track of charts or wasting time searching for a "missing" chart. It also provides easy access to the chart if it is needed while it is out of the office.

When a file is removed, a guide may be placed where the chart is normally filed (Figures 5.10 and 5.11). Medical charts are usually removed from their filing location (for reasons other than a patient visit) only by the physician.

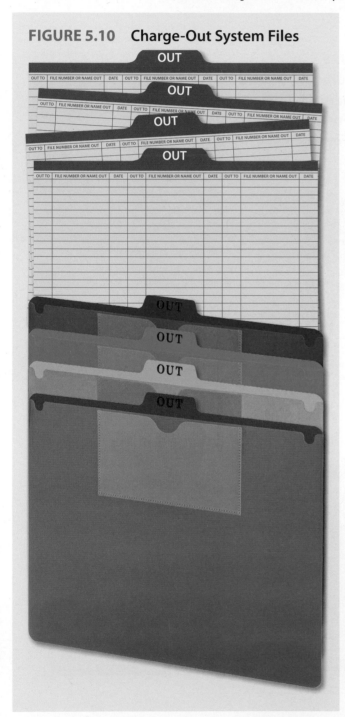

FIGURE 5.10   Charge-Out System Files

FIGURE 5.11   Charge-Out System Form

HEALTH RECORD RECEIPT
FILE CHARGEOUT AND DISPOSITION RECORD

NAME (Last)	(First)	(Middle)

AGE	SEX	SIN

ADDRESS

RECEIVED FROM	DATE

TRANSFERRED TO	DATE

REMARKS

INSTRUCTIONS

This form is designed for use as a permanent record of receipt and disposition of the HEALTH RECORD.

(A) For each HEALTH RECORD received, complete lines 1 through 4 and file in the HEALTH RECORD.

(B) Upon transfer complete line 5 and retain form in permanent files.

(C) Whenever HEALTH RECORD is temporarily removed from files enter information provided for below and retain form in HEALTH RECORD files.

FILE CHARGE-OUT

DATE	RECEIVED BY AND/OR LOCATION

REFERENCES

College of Physicians and Surgeons of Ontario (CPSO). (2000). Policy statement #4-12, "Medical records." http://www .cpso.on.ca/policies-publications/policy/medical-records.

RESOURCES

Medical Records and Health Information Technicians–Career Profile:
http://www.youtube.com/watch?v=PCVNp1PrFM8

ARMA Canada:
http://www.armacanada.org

How to file using terminal digit:
http://www.youtube.com/watch?v=8E48ohvzG_Y

Canadian Electronic Management Record systems or Canadian Electronic Health Record systems

- TelusHealth: http://www.telushealth.com
- OSCAR: http://www.oscarcanada.org
- Nightingale: http://www.nightingalemd.ca
- P&P Data Systems: http://www.p-pdata.com
- QHR Accuro: http://www.qhrtechnologies.com

REVIEW QUESTIONS

True or False?

1. When selecting a filing system, consider security and expansion.

2. In subject filing, items are filed by the topic of the item.

3. The acronym SOAP stands for *Subjective*, *Objective*, *Assessment*, and *Purpose*.

4. One advantage of paper-based filing systems is that they are easy to move.

5. Charge-out guides are used to track employees who have left the office for lunch.

6. All test results should be signed or initialled by the physician before filing in the patient's chart.

Multiple Choice

1. For patient charts, the most common filing system used is
   a. numeric
   b. geographic
   c. alphabetical
   d. subject

2. A chronological filing system
   a. is out of date and frequently used
   b. uses the alphabet to identify and locate patient records
   c. uses numbers
   d. is usually used to file patient records within the patient's chart

3. Which of the following organizations developed the rules for alphabetical filing?
   a. HIPPA
   b. ARMA
   c. CPSO
   d. CMA

4. What is the function of a POMR?
   a. It organizes charts in reverse chronological order.
   b. It organizes charts according to the patient's first visit.
   c. It organizes charts in sections that correspond to the chart components.
   d. It organizes charts in chronological order.

5. Patient information (e.g., test results, referral letters) may be received in
   a. paper format
   b. electronic format
   c. graphic format
   d. all of the above

6. A filing system in which documents are arranged in the chart in sections is known as
   a. SOMR
   b. POMR
   c. alphabetical
   d. SOAP format

7. What is the most important part of any filing system?
   a. the indexing
   b. the coding
   c. the filing
   d. the annotating

8. Which of the following sequences is correctly filed alphabetically?

   a. Jason Smith, Jacob Smythe, Jon Smith, J.A. Smith

   b. J.A. Smith, Jason Smith, Jon Smith, Jacob Smythe

   c. Jason Smith, J.A. Smith, Jon Smith, Jacob Smythe

   d. Jacob Smythe, Jason Smith, J.A. Smith, Jon Smith

9. Choose the correct chart labels for the following (see Appendix 5.1, step 1): Perry T. Le Clair, Peter De La Cruz, Ann McKenzie, Anna MacKenzie, Suzanne Mackenzie, Paul Le Clair.

   a. PTLECL, DELACR, MCK, MACK, MA, PLECL

   b. LEC, DEL, MCK, MAC, MAC, LEC

   c. CL, CR, MCK, MACK, MA, CL

   d. PTLECL, DELACR, MCK, MACK, MAC, PLECL

10. Choose the letter that has the names in correct filing order.

   a. Peter De La Cruz, Perry T. Le Clair, Paul Le Clair, Anna MacKenzie, Suzanne Mackenzie, Ann McKenzie

   b. Paul Le Clair, Perry T. Le Clair, Peter De La Cruz, Anna MacKenzie, Suzanne Mackenzie, Ann McKenzie

   c. Peter De La Cruz, Paul Le Clair, Perry T. LeClair, Anna MacKenzie, Suzanne Mackenzie, Ann McKenzie

   d. Peter De La Cruz, Paul Le Clair, Perry T. LeClair, Suzanne Mackenzie, Anna MacKenzie, Ann McKenzie

Short Answer

1. What is a medical record?

2. What document is attached to the inside front cover of a patient's chart?

3. What is the purpose of colour coding a patient file?

4. What are the advantages and disadvantages of open-shelf filing?

5. Define and explain POMR.

6. How can a medical office administrator protect patient information in the office?

HYBRID LEARNING

1. Find the video "Medical Records and Health Information Technicians—Career Profile" on YouTube and answer the following questions:

   a. Who counts on medical record technicians the most?

   b. What does a medical record technician need to be prepared for?

   c. What does a medical record technician need to pay strict attention to?

2. Visit ARMA Canada's website. Write a summary on how you can become a member and how membership might benefit you.

3. Find the video on how to file using terminal digit on YouTube. Then, write a brief summary explaining the process.

ACTIVITIES

1. Match each filing system to its corresponding description.

   Filing systems

   1 Straight numeric

   2 Terminal digit

   3 Alphabetical

   4 Alphanumeric

   5 Colour coding

   Descriptions

   A can help prevent misfiling

   B one of the oldest and most straightforward systems

   C strict sequential order

   D segments a number into component parts

   E uses a combination of numbers and letters

2. Using the Internet, search for a description of a popular Canadian Electronic Management Record system or a Canadian Electronic Health Record system.

   List the EMR features of at least two sources. How are they similar or different? Which one would you prefer to work with? Explain.

3. Using the source-oriented medical records system, create a table with the following headings: Diagnostic Reports, Progress Reports, Medications, and Laboratory Results. Sort the list of medical documents under the correct heading and in the correct order.

Diagnostic Reports	Progress Reports	Medications	Laboratory Results

Use the following list of medical documents to complete this question and question 4:

List of medical documents:

- Prescription for Maxalt 5-mg wafer, Sept. 12, 2010
- Prescription for Maxalt 10-mg tablet, Oct. 10, 2011
- OGTT results, Jan. 4, 2001
- Mammogram, Oct. 5, 2010
- Physician notes regarding patient's depression symptoms, Feb. 10, 2002
- Thyroid blood test, June 2, 2001
- Physician notes: Patient concerned with frequency of migraines; changing prescription from 5 mg to 10 mg Maxalt tablets, Oct. 10, 2011
- Ultrasound, Mar. 10, 1991
- Prescription for Z-Pak (one 3-day dose pack), Oct. 2, 1979
- CT scan, July 5, 1996

- Chest X-ray, June 12, 1982
- Bone densitometry results, May 12, 2013
- Prescription for Amoxicillin 5 mcg/mL, Jan. 2, 2007
- Physician notes: Discussion regarding recent weight gain and referral to D. Watson, Dietician, Mar. 2, 2002
- FOB test, Aug. 10, 2008
- Physician notes: Patient reporting abdominal pain; requesting MRI scan, Dec. 12, 2009
- MRI abdominal scan, Jan. 5, 2009
- Prescription for Phentermine Oral 30 mg, Jun. 10, 2002
- Mammogram, Oct. 10, 2011
- Prescription for Crestor 20-mg tablets, May 3, 2012

4. Create a new list organizing the medical documents listed above in reverse chronological order.

5. Using the Outguide below, fill in the following information regarding medical records that have been borrowed—the first three by Dr. Gutelius, General Surgeon, KGH 613-465-5588, and the second three by Dr. Smith, GP, Family Medicine 613-542-6847. Make up dates on which the medical record was borrowed and returned.

- James Brown DOB 10/23/1947
- Mary Johnson DOB 8/12/1997
- Yeo-lin Kim DOB 9/2/2002
- Kyle Frances DOB 8/5/1956
- Johannas VanGordon DOB 12/12/2012
- Mary Lou Gains DOB 4/5/1982

OUTGUIDE					
Record (include name and DOB)	Borrower (include contact number or location)	Date	Signature	Return Date and Signature	

6. The following subject file folders and primary guides have been left on your desk. Place each subject folder and primary guide in the correct "drawer" (to the right) and in the correct order:

- Computers
- C Miscellaneous
- Caterers
- Office Supplies
- Subscriptions
- Rent
- A
- R
- O
- C
- S
- Professional Fees
- P
- Q
- Conferences
- Utilities
- HR
- H
- U
- P Miscellaneous

A–E	F–J	K–O	P–T	U–Z

7. Using a table with unit headings, index and alphabetize the following personal names. Write Unit 1 names in all capital letters.

   For example:

NAME	UNIT 1	UNIT 2	UNIT 3	UNIT 4
Senator Robert Ackerman, 3rd	ACKERMAN	Robert	3	Senator

- Alan Shillings
- Anne Smythe
- Andrew Victory
- Chen Lee
- Harry Jack
- Susan A. Williams
- Delilah Jack
- Daneeka Ross
- Jade Kim
- S. Hank Williams
- Victoria A. Anderson
- Elise Van Der Meer
- Kayla O'Neal
- Peter MacDouglas
- Geoff Von Lowe
- Charles Van de Meer
- Lisa McVey
- Wilma LaVoy
- Cindy VanZant
- Virginia McAnderson

- Della McDougal
- Linda Harper-Hoff
- Patricia Wangst
- Sherry-Lynn Acker
- Gina Jones-Acker
- Luke DeJoy
- Joan Wangst-Lu
- Yves Dude-Williams
- Angie-Sue D'Meer
- B.K. Tassle
- S.U. McVey
- K.V. Bander
- Wm. Anderson
- Sgt. Bhupender Singh
- Regina Nourse, MD
- Mrs. Ophelia Acker, PhD
- Princess Diana
- Jeremy A. Finn, III
- Senator Romeo Dallaire
- Sister Regina Acker

8. Using a table with unit headings, index and alphabetize the following business names. Write Unit 1 names in all capital letters.

   For example:

NAME	UNIT 1	UNIT 2	UNIT 3	UNIT 4	UNIT 5
Twelve Points Bar & Grill	TWELVE	Points	Bar	And	Grill

- The Globe and Mail
- Bank of Montreal
- Environmental Lawn Care
- Col. Smart Clothing Accessories
- Lloyds of London Insurance
- El Camino Soccer Group
- St. Martha's Elementary School
- L.B. Golf & Country Club
- CKLC Television
- Kaminer and Kaminer, Attys.
- Kelly Services Agy.
- LuLu Lemon Clothing
- Cunningham-Swan Law Firm
- Dr. Rite Medical Supply Co.

- J&J Towing
- Kingston General Hospital
- Lil' Duck-walk Daycare
- 75th Street Pharmacy
- #1 Auto Body Shop
- $ Saved Used Furniture
- # One Auto Body Shop
- 75th Street Drug Store
- 2nd Hand Thrift Shop
- Second Hand Thrift Shop
- The $ Bargain Bin
- Dollar Pharmacy
- King & King Bookstore
- King & King Attorneys

9. Using the relative index below, file the following subjects:

- BAC Computers
- Hydro One
- Associations
- Jelly 'n' Jam Caterers
- Brothers Plumbing
- Holiday Records
- Commercial Artists
- Computer Techies
- Promotional Products

- Ms. Melissa's Lunchbox
- Day Planners
- Medical Office Administrators Symposium
- Dynacare
- Lemon Electric
- Payroll
- Letterhead
- Staples

- Shopper's Medical Supplies
- Conference Board of Canada
- Leasing Agreement
- Rent Review
- Canadian Medical Laboratories
- Varsity Property Managers
- Danicks Filing Systems
- Premier Medical Supply
- Patient Complaints

FILED UNDER	SUBJECT
Advertising	
Business and Trade Organizations	
Caterers	
Computers	
Conferences	
Contractors	
Human Resources	
Laboratories	
Lease	
Maintenance	
Medical Supplies	
Miscellaneous	
Office Supplies	
Printers	
Utilities	

APPENDIX 5.1

Building the Patient Chart

To create a paper chart, follow the steps below.

STEP 1

At the bottom of the folder end tab, place colour-coded labels that identify the patient.

Options:

- first two letters of last name (see Figure 5.12), or
- first three letters of last name

Note: See ARMA rules regarding prefixes, articles, and hyphens (Appendix 5.2, Rules 2 and 3). These must be incorporated when creating chart labels so that charts are easily accessible.

LaForest = LA or LAF

D'Havilland = DH or DHA

STEP 2

Create two other labels for the outside of the chart:

1. a duplicate label identifying the patient by name and birthdate, and
2. a detailed label with the patient's demographic details.

Label 1: Duplicate Label

VASER, ANN   **8/10/1965**

Label 2: Detailed Patient Information

VASER, ANN
1114 Kensington Boulevard
Kingston ON K7L 2T8
August 10, 1965
Home: 613-555-5555
Work: 613-544-5400

HC# 1234567890

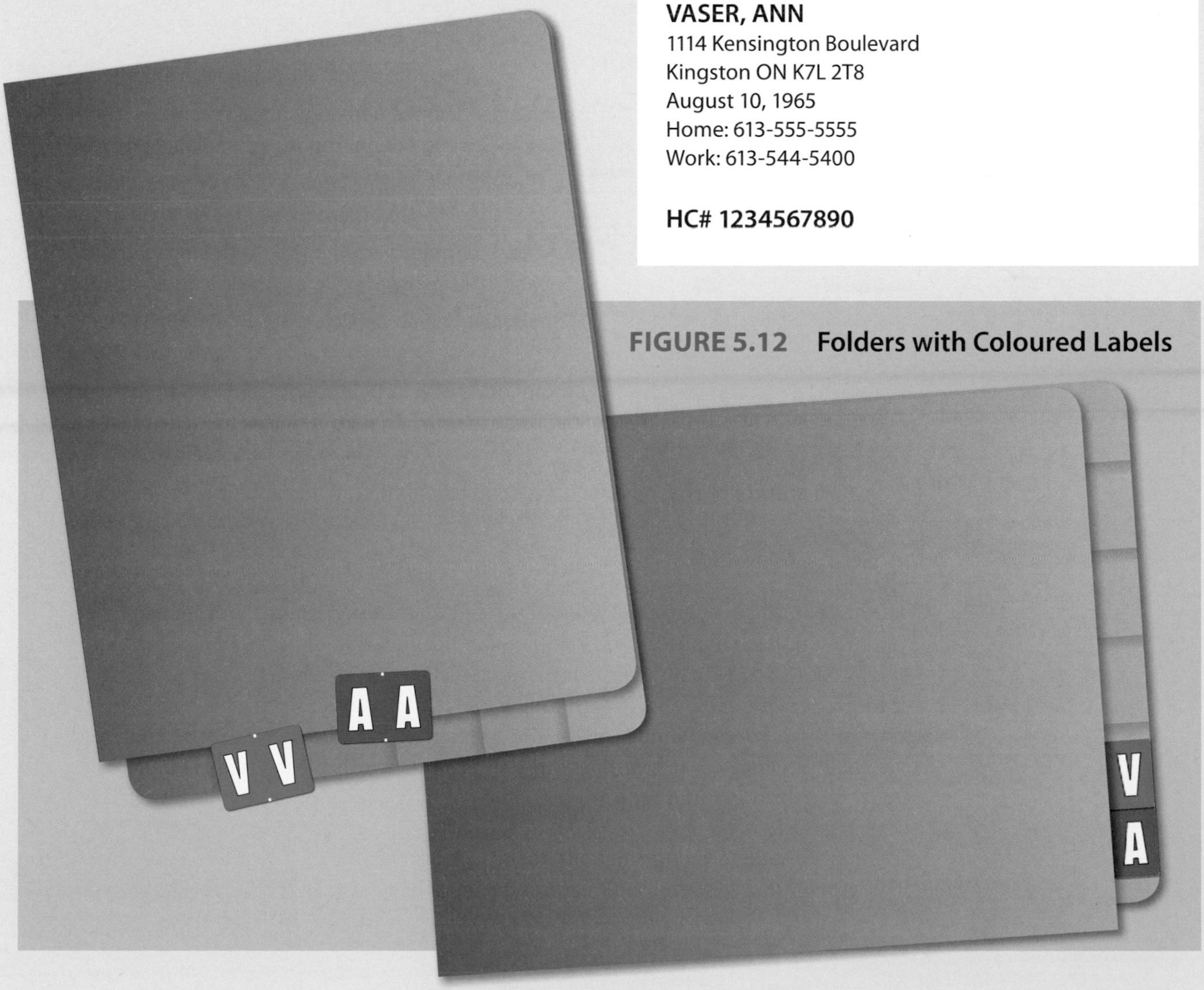

FIGURE 5.12   Folders with Coloured Labels

Place the duplicate label on the folder end tab, above the coloured letters; place the detailed label on the front upper-right corner of the chart. (See Figure 5.13.)

STEP 3

1. Tape (at all four corners) a Problem List to the left inside cover of the chart.
2. Tape (at the two top corners) the Cumulative Profile/Initial Visit to the right inside cover of the chart.
3. Insert (do not tape) a Progress Notes page for the physician to record notes during each visit. (See Figure 5.14.)

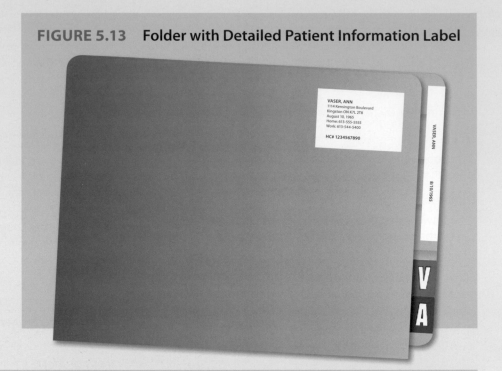

FIGURE 5.13   Folder with Detailed Patient Information Label

FIGURE 5.14   Interior of Folder with Problem List and Progress Notes

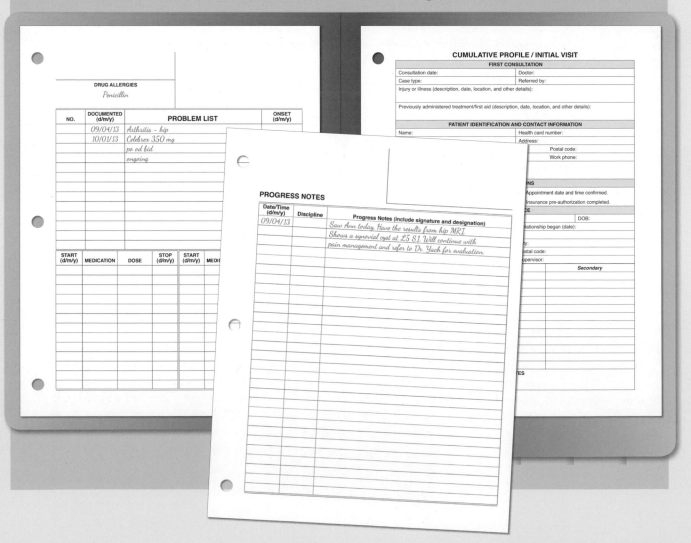

An electronic medical record will contain the same information as the paper chart. Below is an example of an electronic chart.

FIGURE 5.15   Electronic Medical Record

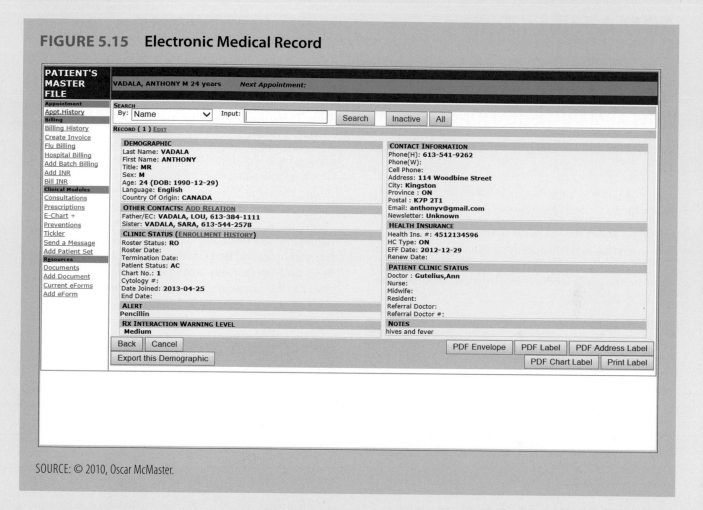

SOURCE: © 2010, Oscar McMaster.

APPENDIX 5.2

ARMA Filing Rules

BASIC FILING RULES CONSISTENT WITH ARMA INTERNATIONAL

To file correctly, the MA must be familiar with the following terms.

Unit—The name or filing label is divided into units. For example, the label "Ann Marie Vadala" has three units.

Indexing—Allows the MA to determine the order of the units in a name, and which name to file a record under. For example, if you are filing by a person's name, the last name would be the key unit or first unit—the unit that the name would be filed under.

Mary Ellen Weigers		
Key Unit	*Second Unit*	*Third Unit*
Weigers	Mary	Ellen

Business:

Shopper's Drug Mart		
Key Unit	*Second Unit*	*Third Unit*
Shoppers	Drug	Mart

Alphabetizing Unit by Unit—The first step in alphabetizing is to alphabetize unit by unit. If the names in Unit 1 are exactly the same, then continue to alphabetize by Unit 2. If the first and second units are the same, the next step is to alphabetize by Unit 3, and so on.

NAME	UNIT 1	UNIT 2	UNIT 3
Sara Julie Hough	Hough	Sara	J
Sara Kate Hough	Hough	Sara	Julie
Sara J Hough	Hough	Sara	Kate

Remember: Nothing comes before something.

THE 12 RULES OF ARMA FILING

Rule 1: Names of Individuals

Individual names are filed last name first—for example, last name goes under Unit 1, first name or initial goes under Unit 2, middle name or initial goes under Unit 3. When indexing the name of an individual, arrange the units in this order: last name as Unit 1, first name or initial as Unit 2, and middle name or initial as Unit 3, and so on. When two names in Unit 1 begin with the same letter, you consider the next or second letter in arranging for alphabetical order. If both the first and second letters are the same, consider the third letter, and so on, until the letters are different.

All punctuation is omitted.

NAME	UNIT 1	UNIT 2	UNIT 3
Becky Adam	ADAM	Becky	
Susan F. Adams	ADAMS	Susan	F
Terri Adams	ADAMS	Terri	
William Ken Jenner	JENNER	William	Ken
William Johnson	JOHNSON	William	
Winifred Jung	JUNG	Winifred	
Frank Schiller	SCHILLER	Frank	
Frank B. Schiller	SCHILLER	Frank	B
Debbie Shirley	SHIRLEY	Debbie	
Ann Marie Weston	WESTON	Ann	Marie
Anna Weston	WESTON	Anna	
David Westonia	WESTONIA	David	

Rule 2: Personal Names with Prefixes, Articles, or Particles

Ignore any apostrophe or space that may appear within or after the prefix.

Commonly used prefixes include *d', D', de, De, Del, De la, Di, Du, El, Fitz, La, Le, Lo, Los, M', Mac, Mc, O', Saint, St., Ste., Te, Ter, Van, Van de, Van der, Von,* and *Von der.*

NAME	UNIT 1	UNIT 2	UNIT 3
Anna D'Elea	DELEA	Anna	
Olivia Dupont	DUPONT	Olivia	
Paul Dupont	DUPONT	Paul	
Charles B. Le Clair	LECLAIR	Charles	B
James A. Macdonald	MACDONALD	James	A
Terry C. McDonald	MCDONALD	Terry	C
Cecelia Van Ness	VANNESS	Cecelia	
John Vanness	VANNESS	John	

Rule 3: Hyphenated Personal Names

Consider a hyphenated first, middle, or last name as one unit. Do not include the hyphen in the unit name.

NAME	UNIT 1	UNIT 2	UNIT 3
Victoria Adams-Rooney	ADAMSROONEY	Victoria	
Jack DaVries	DAVRIES	Jack	
Jack DeVries-Jones	DEVRIESJONES	Jack	
Greg Sean Lee	LEE	Greg	Sean
Greg Sean-Lee	SEANLEE	Greg	
Annie Sean-Lees	SEANLEES	Annie	
Kaya-Lynne S. Shultz	SHULTZ	Kayalynne	S

Rule 4: Single Letters and Abbreviations of Personal Names

Initials in personal names (A.M., M.V.) are considered separate indexing units. Abbreviated personal names (Wm., Al.) and nicknames (Pam, Kate, Alex) are indexed as they are written.

NAME	UNIT 1	UNIT 2	UNIT 3
A.J. Anderson	ANDERSON	A	J
Liz Billings	BILLINGS	LIZ	
Lou Chandler	CHANDLER	LOU	
Wm. Danielson	DANIELSON	WM	
T.J. Sampson	SAMPSON	T	J
Geo. T. Vickory	VICKORY	GEO	T

Rule 5: Personal Names with Titles and Suffixes

Titles (Dr., Prof., Mrs., Ms.) and suffixes (2nd, II, Jr., CPA, PhD) used with a person's name are the last indexing unit. If a name contains both a title and a suffix, the title is the last unit.

Royal and religious titles (King, Princess, Father, Sister) are considered professional designation suffixes and are written as personal names, but if followed by only a given name or a surname (Father Peter, Princess Victoria), they are indexed as written.

NAME	UNIT 1	UNIT 2	UNIT 3	UNIT 4
Susanne Billings, PhD	BILLINGS	Susanne	PhD	
Mrs. Kate Jamieson	JAMIESON	Kate	Mrs	
King Leer	KING	Leer		
Mrs. Trudy Leader	LEADER	Trudy	Mrs	
Ms. Trudy Leader	LEADER	Trudy	Ms	
Sister Mary	SISTER	Mary		
Father Peter Timms	TIMMS	Peter	Father	
Peter M. Trousdale III	TROUSDALE	Peter	M	III
Mr. Alex Ware, Jr.	WARE	Alex	Jr	Mr
Dr. Bob Wild	WILD	Bob	Dr	

Rule 6: Names of Businesses and Organizations

Business names are indexed as written, using their letterhead or trademark as a guide.

In general, *each word* in a business name is a separate unit; however, when "The" is the first word of the business name, it is always the last unit.

NAME	UNIT 1	UNIT 2	UNIT 3	UNIT 4	UNIT 5
A1 Travel Agency	A1	Travel	Agency		
Betty's Bootique	BETTYS	Bootique			
The Coat Factory	COAT	Factory	The		
Coffee and More	COFFEE	And	More		
Coffee Is Us	COFFEE	Is	Us		
Cpt. Bly's Surf & Turf	CPT	Blys	Surf	and	Turf
Doug's U-Hauling	DOUGS	Uhauling			
Dr. Trunk's Tree Remedy	DR	Trunks	Tree	Remedy	
El Ninõ Mexican Restaurant	EL NINO	Mexican	Restaurant		
Kingston Brown Daily News	KINGSTON	Brown	Daily	News	
St. Anthony Lawn Care	STANTHONY	Lawn	Care		
The Ten Dollar Store	TEN	Dollar	Store	The	

Rule 7: Letters and Abbreviations in Business and Organization Names

Single letters in business and organization names are indexed as written. If single letters are separated by spaces, index each letter as a separate unit. An acronym, such as ARMA or L.A.S.E.R., is indexed as one unit regardless of punctuation or spacing.

NAME	UNIT 1	UNIT 2	UNIT 3	UNIT 4
A R C Industries	A	R	C	Industries
ACE Rent A Car	ACE	Rent	A	Car
ARC, Inc.	ARC	Inc		
CBC News	CBC	News		
CKWS Radio Station	CKWS	Radio	Station	
J P Plumbing	J	P	Plumbing	
Me 2U Esthetics	ME	2U	Esthetics	
Spiegel Mfg. Corp.	SPIEGEL	Mfg	Corp	

Rule 8: Punctuation and Possessives in Business and Organization Names

Ignore all punctuation when indexing business and organization names (e.g., commas, periods, hyphens, apostrophes, dashes, exclamation points, question marks, quotation marks).

NAME	UNIT 1	UNIT 2	UNIT 3
A1 Rent-a-Car	A1	Rentacar	
All-for-One Thrift Shop	ALLFORONE	Thrift	Shop
The Eagle's Aery	EAGLES	Aery	The
Indoor/Outdoor Carpeting	INDOOROUTDOOR	Carpeting	
Jam 'n' Jelly Catering	JAMNJELLY	Catering	
The Open Door?	OPEN	Door	The
The Sawmill!	SAWMILL	The	

Rule 9: Numbers in Business and Organization Names

Arabic numbers written in digits (1, 2, 5, 310) and Roman numerals (II, X, M) are considered one unit and are filed in numeric order before alphabetical characters.

Arabic numbers are filed before Roman numerals (5, 310, X, M).

Numbers spelled out (one, twenty, fifty) are filed alphabetically and appear after numbers written in digits or Roman numerals.

Names with numbers included are filed in ascending order (lowest to highest number) before alphabetical names.

The letters *st*, *rd*, and *th* following an Arabic number are ignored (1st is indexed as 1, 2nd as 2, 5th as 5, and so on).

Hyphenated numbers (7-11 Gas Bar) are indexed according to the number before the hyphen, and the number after the hyphen is ignored (7 Gas Bar). An Arabic number followed by a hyphen and a word (7-Stars) is considered one unit (7Stars), and the hyphen is ignored.

NAME	UNIT 1	UNIT 2	UNIT 3	UNIT 4	UNIT 5
1-2-3 Take Out	1	Take	Out		
5 Minutes or Less Esthetics	5	Minutes	Or	Less	Esthetics
12B Batting Club	12B	Batting	Club		
85th Street Plaza	85	Street	Plaza		
4-Day Cruises	4DAY	Cruises			
XXI Forever	XXI	Forever			
Amy's Diner	AMYS	Diner			
B12 Powerhouse	B12	Powerhouse			
Jim's 3-Way Window Washing	JIMS	3Way	Window	Washing	
Jim's Auto Shop	JIMS	Auto	Repair		
Sixty-Nine Steak House	SIXTYNINE	Steak	House		
Twenty Harbour Street Fest	TWENTY	Harbour	Street	Fest	

Rule 10: Symbols in Business and Organization Names

If a symbol is part of a name, the symbol is indexed as if spelled out. When a symbol is used with a number without spacing between ($2, #10), it is considered one unit and the symbol is spelled out (2DOLLAR, NUMBER10).

SYMBOL	INDEXED AS
&	AND
¢	CENT
$	DOLLAR or DOLLARS
#	NUMBER, POUND, or POUNDS
%	PERCENT

NAME	UNIT 1	UNIT 2	UNIT 3	UNIT 4
50¢ Donut Shop	50CENT	Donut	Shop	
Ann's Jewellery House	ANNS	Jewellery	House	
D & D Dye	D	And	D	Dye
$ Days Campgrounds	DOLLAR	Days	Campgrounds	
The Dollar Store	DOLLAR	Store	The	
Every $ Counts Store	EVERY	Dollar	Counts	Store

Rule 11: Government Alphabetizing by Address

If two organizational names are otherwise identical, alphabetize them according to their addresses in this order: city, province/state, street name, direction, street number.

NAME	UNIT 1	UNIT 2	UNIT 3	UNIT 4	UNIT 5	UNIT 6	UNIT 7
St. Lawrence College, 2288 Parkdale Avenue, Brockville, ON	STLAWRENCE	College	Brockville	ON	Parkdale	Avenue	2288
St. Lawrence College, 2 St. Lawrence Drive, Cornwall, ON	STLAWRENCE	College	Cornwall	ON	StLawrence	Drive	2
St. Lawrence College, 25 Johnson Street, Kingston, ON	STLAWRENCE	College	Kingston	ON	Johnson	Street	25
St. Lawrence College, 100 Portsmouth Avenue, Kingston, ON	STLAWRENCE	College	Kingston	ON	Portsmouth	Street	100

Rule 12: Government Names

Federal names—Government of Canada, Unites States Government—must be written on any record to which they apply and make up the first three units (it is easiest to designate a filing cabinet or area to Government of Canada); the fourth and succeeding units are the name of the department or office. "Department of" and "Office of" are transposed when they are part of the official name.

NAME	UNIT 1	UNIT 2	UNIT 3	UNIT 4	UNIT 5	UNIT 6	UNIT 7
Government of Canada Department of Internal Affairs	Government	Of	Canada	Internal	Affairs	Department (of)	
Government of Canada Department of Labour, Human Rights Office	Government	Of	Canada	Labour	Department (of)	Human	Rights
United States Government Department of Consumer Affairs	United	States	Government	Consumer	Affairs	Department (of)	

In the case of state, province, commonwealth, and territory names, the first unit is the name of the state, province, commonwealth, or territory. The succeeding units are the principal words in the name of the office or department. The words "State of," "County of," "City of," "Department of," and so on are often added only if needed for clarity and if they are in the official name.

NAME	UNIT 1	UNIT 2	UNIT 3	UNIT 4	UNIT 5
Alberta Child Health Benefit	ALBERTA	Child	Health	Benefit	
British Columbia Ministry of the Environment	BRITISH COLUMBIA	Environment	Ministry (of the)		
Nova Scotia Department of Agriculture	NOVA SCOTIA	Agriculture	Department (of)		
Nova Scotia Department of Fisheries & Aquaculture	NOVA SCOTIA	Fisheries	And	Aquaculture	Department (of)
Ontario Ministry of Health	ONTARIO	Health	Ministry (of)		
Ontario Home Warranty Program	ONTARIO	Home	Warranty	Program	

Foreign government names are indexed first by the English name of the foreign country, then by the name of the department, ministry, bureau, and so on.

NAME	UNIT 1	UNIT 2	UNIT 3	UNIT 4	UNIT 5
Principat d'Andorra/Principality of Andorra	ANDORRA	Principality	of		
Federal Republic of Germany	GERMANY	Federal	Republic	of	
Republic of Bharat	BHARAT	Republic	of		
Department of Human Resources Brazil	BRAZIL	Human	Resources	Department	of

Sources: Appendix 5.2 is based on data from *The Gregg Reference Manual*, by W. Sabin, 2010, McGraw-Hill; "The 12 Rules of Filing (Information Organization and Management)," University of Idaho; and *Records Management*, by D. West, 2002, St. Paul, MN: Paradigm.

Scheduling

6

LEARNING OUTCOMES

After completing this chapter, you should be able to:

- identify the types of scheduling for patient appointments
- explain the guidelines for determining the order and length of patient appointments
- schedule and monitor appointments
- explain the importance of screening in scheduling appointments
- identify and use abbreviations associated with scheduling
- understand how to maintain confidentiality in scheduling appointments (by computer and manually)
- schedule patients in both manual and computerized systems

Time stays long enough for anyone who will use it.

—Leonardo Da Vinci

Introduction

As a medical office administrator (MA), you will need to know how to schedule appointments. Scheduling patient appointments is a common daily procedure within every type of medical office, and scheduling appointments efficiently and effectively is an important skill.

Successfully managing appointments and patient flow is one of the most challenging administrative tasks. When scheduling is done correctly, the physician's office will run more smoothly and efficiently—patients will have shorter wait times, and staff (physicians and office administrators) will be less stressed.

Types of Scheduling

The type of medical office, the **physician's appointment preferences**, and patient demographics contribute to the type of scheduling chosen.

MAs answer incoming phone calls and schedule patients according to the physician's availability. The scheduling system may involve a pen-and-paper calendar, but is more likely to involve computerized scheduling software.

A paper appointment calendar can be time-consuming. Time is lost searching through pages to find an open appointment time; the appointment details must be handwritten and are often difficult to read because of messy handwriting and double bookings or appointment changes that are squeezed into a single time slot on the calendar. A paper appointment calendar also can be easily destroyed. Eraser marks or a coffee spill can blur appointments. Today, it is rare to find an office that books appointments in a paper calendar. However, the biggest motivator to switch to scheduling software is billing. Provincial billing procedure requires electronic submissions of billing information. Booking with only paper scheduling would add significant time to the MA's task of submitting billing.

Today, most offices have web-based electronic medical record (EMR) software. These practice management systems usually work with Windows and Apple computers and offer scheduling, billing, and accounting capabilities to help keep the medical office running efficiently. An EMR software matrix also allows the user to manage multiple physicians, block times, set appointment types, and other preferences to meet the needs of individual offices. EMRs allow the MA to back up appointments so that appointment information is not lost. Colour-coding the appointments helps MAs easily see types of appointments booked, and electronic records permit tracking and collecting of information for research.

The MA should be aware that there are nine basic types of scheduling.

DID YOU KNOW?

Effective January 1, 2003, physicians or medical laboratories registering for the first time with the Ministry of Health and Long-Term Care were required to submit claims via electronic data transfer (EDT). If they continued to use a health claim card, the ministry charged physicians for each submission. This effectively encouraged physicians to use EMR software.

1. Fixed Office Hours

Fixed office hours, also called "open scheduling" or "stream scheduling," is probably the most common type of scheduling. An office is open for fixed hours (e.g., 9:00 a.m. to 12 noon and then from 1:30 p.m. to 4:00 p.m.), and patients are seen in a steady stream, at previously booked appointment times. Appointment time slots are divided into 15-minute segments. Patients who need a 30-minute appointment are given two time slots; patients who need a 45-minute appointment are given three time slots, and so on.

2. Wave Scheduling

In **wave scheduling**, patients are scheduled in the first half hour of every hour. So, if a patient is normally seen every 15 minutes, or "four per" (hour), four patients are scheduled at 9:00 a.m. and are seen on first-come, first-seen basis. As long as some patients arrive early, some late, and some are a no-show, this system works quite well. However, if all patients arrive for their appointment at 9:00 a.m., some of the patients could have as long as a 45-minute wait. When this happens, patients, administrative staff, and physicians become frustrated, and the atmosphere in the office becomes tense.

3. Modified Wave Scheduling

In a **modified wave scheduling** system, two patients are scheduled at 9:00 a.m. and two patients are scheduled at 9:30 a.m. This method ensures a more consistent patient flow than a strict wave scheduling system.

4. Cluster Scheduling/Affinity Scheduling

Cluster scheduling groups similar types of appointments together at specific times and on specific days. For example, all physical examinations might be booked in the morning only, and only on Mondays, Wednesdays, and Fridays. Some physicians prefer to have all of the same kind of complaints scheduled together. They find it easier for scheduling and a more efficient way to see patients.

5. Double Booking

Double booking, which is rarely used as a primary scheduling method, is a form of scheduling when two or more patients are given the same appointment time. This method may be used when there are two or more physicians working at a clinic at one time and each patient is being seen by a different physician. General practitioners commonly use this method to accommodate patients who need to be seen only for a "quick check," or those who require urgent care. For example, a patient who thinks she might have a urinary tract infection might be double booked with a patient being seen for an earache.

It is important for the MA to be aware of the history of both patients—their ages, physical well-being, and problem histories. Very young children and seniors do not make good candidates for double booking, as they often require more time, regardless of the reason for their visit.

Double booking is a skill developed while working in the field, as the office administrator must be familiar with the physician's practices and patient dynamics.

6. Combination or Blended Scheduling

Combination scheduling mixes two types of scheduling. The types most commonly blended or combined are the open/stream scheduling method and the cluster scheduling method.

2. Search for a YouTube video using the key words "YouTube" and "difficult patient." Watch the video on how to deal with patients in a medical office, and provide your thoughts on how this situation was handled. Would you have handled it differently? Explain.

3. When booking appointments, we often interact with patients who have a variety of disabilities, such as hearing, mobility, mental, or verbal disabilities. Conduct an online search on one such disability, and provide a point-form list of techniques that may help you interact with such a patient more effectively.

ACTIVITIES

1. Review the following complaint list. Using Appendix 6.2: Manual Schedule Sheet (or a computer scheduler, if you prefer), decide on the appropriate time period for each appointment. Your physician, Dr. Vinayek Patel, works from 9:00 a.m. to 4:00 p.m. Block off lunch, which is from noon to 1:30 p.m. Dr. Patel will complete general annual exams only in the morning, and likes to complete blood pressure checks between 9:00 a.m. and 10:00 a.m. Use today's date.

APPT. NO.	TIME	LAST NAME	FIRST NAME	DOB	HEALTH CARD NUMBER	PHONE NUMBER	REASON FOR VISIT
1		CUNDALL	Rosie	7/3/1947	7439280002	613-431-6568	Has a boil on her arm
2		FAN	Nu	3/7/1937	7108913527	613-556-0041	Has been experiencing severe dizziness when lying down and then standing up
3		BAMFORD	Annabelle	10/21/1945	3561306635	613-551-3143	Excruciating pain in her left thigh
4		FOURNIER	Arthur	4/11/1942	2760330015	613-548-7514	BP check
5		BANG	Li Hua	5/20/2012	7700722966	613-431-7249	Has had diarrhea x 3 days
6		PORTER	Jack	7/16/2010	5477706895	613-431-6337	Has an earache
7		BALEWA	Adanna	10/22/1990	1820749758	613-431-9805	Has had a cold; she now has a fever and is having trouble getting her breath
8		NORRIS	James	3/29/1971	2908442419	613-551-3163	GA (general annual examination)
9		GARBER	Kendra	6/16/1995	3365242253	613-431-8026	Pain in her lower back
10		ADACHI	Akio	7/27/2008	8482411002	613-431-8232	Vomiting x 3 days
11		FRANKCOM	Kendra	8/9/2004	8249447307	613-431-7819	GA
12		DRURY	Anthony	9/3/1981	7669355589	613-431-7169	Has large sores in mouth
13		GAUDER	Janie	9/11/2000	8625810639	613-431-8079	Possibly has strep throat
14		MOUSALLY	Jammal	6/24/1960	1267526647	613-551-3170	BP check
15		JESSIE	Sue	6/25/1997	9273791446	613-431-7544	GA
16		DUNN	Chuck	10/14/2009	5569472717	613-431-7218	Booked to have stitches removed from right hand
17		MAWAR	Nor	5/28/2011	4834863933	613-551-3160	Possible sore throat, child is cranky and not eating
18		HALL	Sarah	4/20/1986	3666282978	613-431-6509	First prenatal visit
19		PAGET	Walter	10/19/1976	2740149308	613-551-3581	Has a bunion on his left toe
20		FERGUS	Ken	3/21/1990	7857444249	613-431-7587	Has a swollen left testicle
21		DUFF	Hanna	6/08/1989	5421298546	613-542-9874	Pap
22		LANG	Ted	4/06/1998	6874128945	613-572-9854	Needs an allergy shot
23		DUFF	Hilary	5/09/2001	7851235489	613-555-3245	Strep throat

2. Place the following list of sample appointments in priority order by indicating whether they should be referred to the emergency room (ER) or whether they can be booked to see the family physician if the appointment is considered "urgent," "moderate," or "non-urgent."

Priority Order	Patient Is Reporting...
	Minor chest pain
	Prescription renewal for birth control—runs out next week
	Swelling in the ankles—8 months pregnant
	Showing signs of jaundice in the eyes
	Severe sunburn
	Allergic reaction to a bee sting 10 minutes ago
	Infant is coughing and has a fever
	Needs third part of hepatitis C shot
	Feeling depressed for the last week—requesting a counselling appointment
	Requesting a doctor's note for being off sick with the flu
	Has either broken or severely sprained ankle
	Middle-aged woman reports that she fainted
	Well-baby check
	Bleeding from a cut on the leg; applied pressure is not stopping the bleeding
	Rash from camping

3. The following appointments have been scheduled for today. You pulled the charts last night. As you are setting up for the day, you play back the voicemail and have the following messages. All the patients requesting an appointment must be seen today. You will note on the following schedule that the doctor is either out of office or not booking patients at certain times of the day. Use the appointment time guide to schedule the appointments. Be prepared to explain reasons for booking choices. When booking, consider the following:

- Should any of the appointments be referred to the emergency department?
- Are you able to double book any of the appointments?
- Does the type of appointment best suit the morning or the afternoon?

Phone Call 1 Leanne Tyler calls; she would like an appointment for her infant, Tyler. He has diarrhea: 613-389-8521.

Phone Call 2 Cheryl White-Smith calls in a panic; while working in her lab, she spilled some acid on her arm: 613-544-1258

Phone Call 3 Jane Albany—laryngitis: 613-544-6521

Phone Call 4 Kim Cantrell needs an allergy shot: 613-384-5599

Phone Call 5 Shelley Jones has stomach pain—has had pain for past 24 hours, and it is progressively worse: 613-544-7800

Phone Call 6 Charlene McDonald—BP check: 613-542-8923

Phone Call 7 Joe Rogers—BP check: 613-384-1759

Physician: Vadala, Ann				
Time	Patient's Name	Phone	DOB	Reason for Visit
09:00	Smith, Jennifer	613-542-5825	15-06-1995	Flu Shot
09:15				
09:30	Jones, Brittany	613-548-7894	27-01-1985	LN (liquid nitrogen treatment)
09:45				
10:00				
10:15				
10:30				
10:45	Rogers, Tara	613-544-8010	13-07-1997	Pap
11:00				
11:15				
11:30				
11:45				
12:00–13:30		LUNCH		
13:30				
13:45	DO NOT BOOK 13:30–14:00			
14:00				
14:15	Johnson, Rose	613-548-7413	02-03-1990	Tetanus shot
14:30				
14:45				
15:00				
15:15	Henley, Lisa	613-542-6894	02-02-1980	4-wk check for triplets
15:30				
15:45				
16:00				
16:15				
16:30				

APPENDIX 6.1

Appointment Card

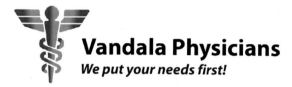

Vandala Physicians
We put your needs first!

400 West Georgia Street
Kingston, ON K6M 3T4
(613) 224-2308

_____

Has an appointment with

_____

Clinical Specialist

_____

Date

_____ a.m.   _____ p.m.

Please give 24 hours' notice of any cancellation
or charges may apply.
Thank you.

APPENDIX 6.2

Manual Schedule Sheet

Appt. No.	Time	Patient's Last Name	Patient's First Name	DOB	Health Card Number	Telephone Number	Reason for Visit
	9:00–9:15						
	9:15–9:30						
	9:30–9:45						
	9:45–10:00						
	10:00–10:15						
	10:15–10:30						
	10:30–10:45						
	10:45–11:00						
	11:00–11:15						
	11:15–11:30						
	11:30–11:45						
	11:45–12:00						
	12:00–12:15						
	12:15–12:30						
	12:30–12:45						
	12:45–1:00						
	1:00–1:15						
	1:15–1:30						
	1:30–1:45						
	1:45–2:00						
	2:00–2:15						
	2:15–2:30						
	2:30–2:45						
	2:45–3:00						
	3:00–3:15						
	3:15–3:30						
	3:30–3:45						
	3:45–4:00						
	4:00–4:15						
	4:15–4:30						

Diagnostics, Medical Imaging, and Common Medical Tests

7

LEARNING OUTCOMES

After completing this chapter, you should be able to:

- describe the role of diagnostic tests in patient care
- discuss the responsibilities of the medical office administrator with respect to diagnostic tests and procedures
- demonstrate how to fill in requisitions with the required information
- explain how to educate clients about laboratory and diagnostic tests
- discuss the procedures involved when test results arrive at the office

Whatever we well understand we express clearly, and words flow with ease.

—Nicholas Boileau

Introduction

A medical office administrator's role focuses on clerical tasks. However, there are situations where the role involves some clinical tasks—for example, in the case of patient tests. As an MA, you should have an understanding of how common tests are performed and how the results of these tests relate to patient care. Clinical tasks that you may be asked to carry out include assisting the physician during a Pap test, completing a urinalysis, taking height and weight measurements, determining body mass index (BMI), and processing laboratory results.

When requested by the physician, a medical office administrator may also take a patient's medical history, educate patients about types of imaging or diagnostic testing, and help patients prepare for tests. In addition, he or she may collect any specimen samples from the patient for lab testing before the exam begins in order to expedite the examination process. An MA will also gather test results, such as blood, tissue, or specimen samples, from laboratories.

Overview of Testing Procedures

Each diagnostic procedure used by the physician—a symptom, sign, or laboratory or radiological examination—deepens the physician's understanding of the patient's illness or disease. Such procedures may provide a conclusive reason for the patient's complaint; even if they do not, they will rule out certain conditions and allow the physician to provide the patient with the best possible care.

BOX 7.1 | Test Results

Part of the MA's role is to review incoming test results. The MA is *definitely not* the final interpreter of test results; however, MAs who can recognize abnormal results will be able to draw these to the physician's attention. The MA can pull the chart when presenting lab results rather than add this step after the physician has reviewed the days' exam findings. What if the physician is away, or out of office for a few days? This could mean treatment delays for the patient. The best MA will be able to keep the physician or the physician's locum informed.

Physicians make decisions about patient care based on clinical information, such as the patient's history and the results of a physical examination; however, this information is not always sufficient to make a diagnosis. When more information is required, the physician may turn to **diagnostic tests**. Diagnostic tests are done to confirm or deny that a patient has a particular condition. They can be performed on every part of the body and can help diagnose many conditions and diseases, including cancer, diabetes, thyroid problems, sexually transmitted diseases, hepatitis, and bacterial and viral infections. For psychiatric conditions, diagnostic tests include psychological and clinical laboratory examinations, as well as brain imaging.

For example, consider a patient who is seen by her general practitioner (GP). She complains of hip/back pain and tingling in her calf, ankle, and foot. The pain is severe and limits mobility. After examination, the physician feels sure that the patient has a slipped disc. The physician prescribes medication and physiotherapy, which may slide the disc back into place. To ensure that the diagnosis is correct, the physician orders magnetic resonance imaging (MRI); this will show whether there is any chance of putting the disc back into place. However, the MRI does not show a slipped disc, but a spinal synovial cyst. This unexpected revelation will change the course of the patient's treatment.

In this example, the physician's diagnosis was proved incorrect by the diagnostic test, and the course of treatment was adjusted to fit this more complete knowledge.

In addition to diagnostic tests, physicians perform screening tests. Unlike diagnostic tests, screening tests are administered to patients who are not showing symptoms of a condition but where risk factors exist, such as a family history of a particular condition. For example, a patient who has no symptoms of cardiovascular disease might have his cholesterol levels measured regularly, particularly if his parents or siblings are experiencing evidence of cardiovascular disease.

DID YOU KNOW?

Newborns are screened for an enzyme that is needed for normal growth and development. The test is known as the phenylketonuria (PKU) test.

Screening tests can detect a range of conditions and illnesses, such as cancers, diabetes, high cholesterol, high blood pressure, and osteoporosis. Amniocentesis is a test administered to women during pregnancy in cases where there is a higher risk of developmental abnormalities, and genetic testing is used to determine whether an individual has a gene for a particular disorder, such as age-related macular degeneration. If a screening test shows that a patient may have a particular condition, a diagnostic test will be done to confirm this.

Medical screening and diagnostic tests include the following:

- blood and urine tests
- analysis of other body fluids
- imaging of the body using **radiology**, MRI, computed tomography (CT), positron emission tomography (PET), angiography, or ultrasonography
- endoscopy, which involves using a camera attached to a tube to observe body cavities, such as the mouth, nose, or intestines
- biopsies, which involve the microscopic examination of samples of tissue that have been removed from a part of the body

See the appendices at the end of this chapter for sample test requisitions.

DID YOU KNOW?

Blood and urine tests are the most common screening and diagnostic tools used by family physicians or general practitioners (GPs).

In general, diagnostic tests are riskier and more expensive than screening tests. They are used in the following situations:

- to prove a diagnosis in symptomatic patients
- to check for disease (as in mammography for women over 50)
- to provide prognostic information for those with established disease (e.g., blood work after cancer therapy to determine the levels of ca125, a protein made by cells in the

body that is found in higher-than-normal amounts in the blood of women with ovarian cancer)

- to monitor therapy (looking at side effects or benefits of a certain treatment)
- to prove that a person is free from disease (e.g., a Pap test to prove the absence of cancer cells)

Before a physician orders a diagnostic test, he or she must consider the benefits of the test against the potential costs and possible adverse effects. Some tests carry a risk. For example, amniocentesis carries a risk of miscarriage, and for this reason, the test is offered only to those who are at greatest risk. The physician is responsible for informing patients of the possible consequences that may flow from discovering the information (e.g., in the case of amniocentesis, being faced with the decision of whether to discontinue the pregnancy).

SCENARIO 7.1

You work as an MA in a medical office. One day, a patient calls to ask for the results of his recent blood work. You have just finished placing this patient's results on the physician's desk and are aware that he has tested positive for a sexually transmitted disease. How will you handle the call?

SCENARIO 7.2

Your physician is away from the office but has left a contact number, to be used only if necessary. You are in the office sorting through test results delivered this morning. You realize that a patient's international normalized ratio (INR) and prothrombin time (PT) values have significantly altered from her last blood work. Considering the patient's test results, should you contact the physician?

Patient Preparation for Tests Requested by the GP

When a GP requests a test for a patient, the MA will often fill out the requisition and discuss the preparatory procedure with the patient.

For example, if the GP requests a colonoscopy for a patient, the MA will fill in the requisition and fax it to the endoscopy clinic. The clinic will then phone the patient to let him or her know the date and time of the test. A colonoscopy requires specific preparation to be effective, and it is important that the patient be clear on what is required. The MA will both organize the paperwork and review with the patient instructions on how to prepare.

See Chapter 4 (Medical Records 1: Legal Framework and Requirements) and Chapter 5 (Medical Records 2: Chart Components, Organization, and Filing Systems) for more information on manual and electronic medical records.

Blood Work

Blood work is one of the most common tests performed. A blood test can give the physician an overall view of the patient's health and highlight areas of concern.

Blood work may be requisitioned to monitor a condition or treatment. In addition, when a patient is seen for a physical examination (general annual health exam), the following two standard blood tests are recommended to establish his or her overall health:

1. the **complete blood count (CBC)**
2. a **chemistry panel**

A CBC counts the number of red blood cells, the different types of white blood cells, and platelets in blood. It also measures hemoglobin and hematocrit levels. An increase or decrease in blood counts will alert the physician to a possible change in the patient's health status. A number of tests fall under the "chemistry panel" umbrella—depending on the type of panel, these tests may assess electrolyte balance, protein, cholesterol, or other chemicals that indicate vascular, kidney, and liver status. For more information and optimal ranges, see Appendix 7.14: Optimal Ranges for Common Blood Tests.

Having blood taken requires that a needle be inserted in the large vein inside the elbow (the most common route), or alternatively, on the dorsal surface of the hand, in the neck, the heel (for infants), and sometimes, the skull. The prick will feel similar to a flu shot or insect sting. Once the needle is inserted, one or more vials will be pushed onto the back of the needle, and when the required amount of blood is in the vial and all vials needed have been taken, the needle will be removed and pressure will be applied for about one minute to the puncture site. When the **phlebotomist**, a medical professional specializing in the drawing of blood for medical tests, is sure that bleeding has stopped from the site, a band-aid will be applied. In order to prevent a recurrence of bleeding from the puncture site, the patient will be asked not to lift anything heavy using that arm for 6 to 8 hours.

No preparation is required for either a CBC or a chemistry panel. However, for a fasting blood test (fasting blood sugar [FBS], fasting triglycerides [cholesterol], fasting lipids [cholesterol and heart disease], and glucose tolerance [diabetes]), individuals must fast (refrain from eating) for 8 to 12 hours before the test.

Imaging

There are four key categories for **imaging**:

1. nuclear medicine (e.g., MRI, bone scan, thyroid scan and thyroid uptake, electrocardiography [ECG/EKG])
2. X-ray (e.g., bone densitometry, mammography, lower gastrointestinal [GI] tract, upper GI tract)
3. ultrasonography (e.g., pelvic, transvaginal, abdominal, obstetrical, breast imaging)
4. CT (e.g., total body scan, virtual colonoscopy/colonography CT)

As an MA, you will be expected to direct the patient to the correct facility and answer questions regarding the procedure, including preparation.

Table 7.1 at the end of this chapter lists the most common screening and diagnostic tests requested by GPs. Many other tests are available, and you may need to become familiar with them over the course of your career. Sample requisition forms are included in the appendices at the end of this chapter.

Patient Preparation for Tests Completed by a GP

Table 7.2 at the end of this chapter lists the most common tests completed by a GP. These tests are administered in the office and provide the GP with an indication of the patient's condition. A Pap test, urinalysis, weight and height, and eye exam are all tests that an office administrator might carry out or assist with. For example, an MA may join the patient and physician in the examining room during a Pap test. The MA will assist by handing the slide and swabs to the physician and then taking the samples for labelling and directing to the appropriate lab. (Note: Owing to the sensitive nature of this and similar exams, a physician should always include a third person for the protection of both the patient and the physician. Physicians should also consider having a parent or guardian, or other third party, present for any examinations of patients who are minors.)

BOX 7.2   Third-Party Presence

"Professional regulators and medico-legal societies are increasingly urging that physicians ensure a third party is present during sensitive procedures, as much for their own protection from allegations of impropriety as to put patients at ease."

SOURCE: "Who Should Be Privy to Your Privates?" by Lauren Vogel, 2012, *Canadian Medical Association Journal*.

See Chapter 3: The Medical Office Environment for more information about the supplies required in a medical office.

SCENARIO 7.3

Ann, an MA, was assisting the doctor with a Pap test. As she was carrying the completed smear to her desk to complete the requisition and prepare the smear for pickup from the lab, the slide slipped out of its container and fell on the rug.

What should Ann do in this situation? Is the smear compromised? If so, how would you approach the patient to explain that the Pap test must be repeated?

SCENARIO 7.4

The physician has requested that the patient have an occult stool test. Upon leaving the office, the patient confides in you that he finds the idea of obtaining samples of stool disgusting and probably won't do it. How can you demonstrate the importance of the test to the patient? Is there any guidance you can offer to ease his disgust and convince him to complete the requested test?

Incoming Laboratory Results

Charting of a patient's health record includes all information regarding the patient's care—encounter notes, prescriptions, allergies, and test results. The MA must ensure that patient charts are up to date so that the physician may provide good-quality and continuity of care; if a chart is not up to date, it will be difficult for the physician to provide the appropriate care.

A working knowledge of incoming test results is essential if the MA is to provide proper support for the physician. It is the responsibility of the MA to ensure that all test results are reviewed by the physician before they are filed, and that they are filed appropriately in each patient's chart. After the physician has reviewed the charts and left a mark (initials, symbol) indicating that the results have been reviewed, the MA may replace the results in the patients'

PRACTICE TIP

When the MA assists the physician with a Pap or other test, he or she should respect the patient's privacy and position him- or herself close enough in order to hand swabs or slides to the physician but angled so that the MA sees little or none of the area being examined. Assisting the physician affords the MA a good opportunity to help the patient relax by adjusting the pillow, making sure the patient is as comfortable as possible, and possibly chatting about the patient's family or other interests.

charts. The MA must pay close attention to any instructions the physician may have written on the test results. For example, the physician may request a follow-up appointment or a change in medication, and the instruction must be dealt with before the result is filed in the chart.

In the past, the term "normal range" was used to describe normal test results; today, it is rarely used because it may be misleading. If a patient's results are outside the range for that test, this does not automatically mean the result is abnormal. Therefore, today the terms "reference range," "reference values," "reference intervals," or "optimal range" are considered more appropriate.

Blood Work Test Results

Blood work is one of the most common test results dealt with in a GP's office. When blood test results are returned to the office, the MA is the first person to review them. If there are several results outside the optimal range, the report should be brought to the physician's immediate attention.

Appendix 7.14 lists the optimal ranges for results of common blood tests.

Thyroid blood tests are also regularly performed to determine how well a patient's thyroid gland is functioning. The blood tests are known as T3, T4, and TSH. Changes in these levels could indicate hypothyroidism or hyperthyroidism.

When a patient has a BMI result that places him or her in the obese category, an **oral glucose tolerance test (OGTT)** may be performed to determine if the patient has diabetes. This blood test generally lasts about two hours, and the patient must have fasted for 10 to 12 hours prior to the test. When the patient arrives, the nurse takes a fasting blood sample and then gives the patient a concentrated glucose drink that must be consumed in a five-minute period. A basic OGTT will take another blood sample two hours later. Depending on the test, other samples may be taken periodically. The patient is considered diabetic if the fasting rate is over 7.0 mmol/L and if the two-hour fasting result is over 7.8 mmol/L.

Patients who have recently had surgery (particularly orthopedic surgery) are prescribed a blood thinner, such as warfarin (Coumadin), to ensure correct clotting times, and to avoid blood clots and deep vein thrombosis (DVT). The frequency and length of time the patient is medicated depend on the type of surgery and the type of anticoagulation therapy used. Clotting time is measured using three tests: **prothrombin time (PT)**, **partial thromboplastin time (PTT)**, and **international normalized ratio (INR)**.

Prothrombin Time Blood Test

This test evaluates the blood for its ability to clot. It is often done before surgery to determine how likely the patient is to have a bleeding or clotting problem during or after surgery.

Normal PT values are between 10 and 12 seconds (results can vary slightly from lab to lab). Common causes of a prolonged PT include vitamin K deficiency; hormone drugs, including hormone replacements and oral contraceptives; disseminated intravascular coagulation (a serious clotting problem that requires immediate intervention); liver disease; and the use of the anti-coagulant drug warfarin. Additionally, the PT result can be altered by a diet high in vitamin K, liver, green tea, dark green vegetables, and soybeans.

Partial Thromboplastin Time Blood Test

This test is performed primarily to determine whether heparin (blood thinning) therapy is effective. It can also be used to detect the presence of a clotting disorder. It does not show the effects of drugs called "low molecular weight heparin," most commonly referred to by the brand name Lovenox.

PRACTICE TIP

If in doubt, find out. Do not guess or assume if you are unsure of test results or correct directions to give a patient. ASK.

PRACTICE TIP

Although as an MA it is your responsibility to bring abnormal blood work results to the physician's attention, the test results from the lab will often clearly indicate which values are outside the "normal range."

Normal PTT values are between 30 and 45 seconds (results can vary slightly from lab to lab). Extended PTT times can be a result of anticoagulation therapy, liver problems, lupus, and other diseases that result in poor clotting.

International Normalized Ratio Blood Test

This test is used to ensure that the results from a PT test are the same at one lab as they are at another. In the 1980s, the World Health Organization determined that patients might be at risk because the results of a PT test could vary from one lab to another, based upon the way the test was done. The "normal" range for one lab would be different from a "normal" value from another lab, creating problems for patients who were being treated in several locations. In order to standardize the results among labs, the INR was created. The INR result should be the same, regardless of where the tests are performed.

Normal INR values range from 1 to 2.

While there is no set timetable for blood testing of patients taking blood thinners, patients will typically be tested from every two or three days to once a week until levels are stable, then may progress to testing twice a month. INR, PPT, and PT results are often reported to the office administrator verbally. When these values are reported, they must be brought immediately to the physician's attention because the patient's drug dosage must often be adjusted to secure optimal ranges.

Pap Test Results

In Ontario, physicians are allowed to perform Pap tests once every 36 months on females between the ages of 21 and 65, as long as their last three Pap tests have been normal. If the patient has an abnormal test result, the lab will request that a repeat Pap test be performed in six weeks to one year, depending on the findings.

When an MA receives a Pap test result that requires a follow-up Pap test, he or she should bring this to the physician's attention, then follow through with a phone call to the patient and an appointment booking. For sample results, see Appendix 7.15: Pap Test Results.

Urine Test Results

If a urine sample is sent to a lab for further testing, the lab will test the sample for protein, glucose, ketones, and red and white blood cells, and the returned requisition will clearly show any concerns about the functioning of the patient's urinary system. Abnormal values may indicate a urinary tract infection, kidney damage, high blood pressure, diabetes, kidney stones, or other problems of the urinary system.

If results are abnormal, the physician will prescribe appropriate medication and ask the office administrator to call the patient and inform him or her of the need to fill a prescription and to book a follow-up appointment. Other types of abnormal results may require a referral to a urologist for a more in-depth evaluation. The office administrator is responsible for booking the follow-up.

TABLE 7.1   Common Screening and Diagnostic Tests

NUCLEAR MEDICINE IMAGING TECHNIQUES

Safe, painless techniques that use small amounts of radiopharmaceuticals (radioactive compounds used for diagnostic or therapeutic purposes) to diagnose and treat disease. Special cameras and computers produce very precise images of particular parts of the body.

For sample requisitions, see Appendix 7.1: General Imaging Requisition and Appendix 7.2: Nuclear Medicine Requisition.

Imaging Technique	About the Test	What to Expect	Preparation
Magnetic resonance imaging (MRI) *For a sample requisition, see Appendix 7.3: MRI Requisition.*	• Detailed, cross-sectional images of body organs and tissues are produced by a magnetic field and radio waves passing through the body.	• The MRI unit is a large, tube-shaped magnet. Patients must remove all metal and magnetic objects from their person before the exam. • The machine produces loud noises while running, and headphones are provided to help dampen the noise. An emergency call button is also provided, should the patient become claustrophobic or otherwise need to use it. • Patients must remain completely still, as any movement may skew the results.	None required.
Bone scan	• Used to diagnose and monitor various types of bone disease and injury, including infection and cancer that has spread from an organ to the bone.	• A small amount of radiopharmaceutical is injected into an arm vein. Imaging can occur immediately, in a few minutes or hours, or days after radiopharmaceutical injection. There is no radiation from the camera. • Imaging typically takes 15–20 minutes (up to one hour) and requires the patient to lie very still while a camera moves above and around his or her body. If the images aren't clear the first time, additional pictures may be required. • Following the scan, women who are breastfeeding will need to discard their milk and use formula for 1–2 days to ensure that the radioactive tracer has left the body before they resume breastfeeding.	Usually, none required. However, patients should be asked whether they have, in the last 4 days, had an X-ray test using barium contrast material or taken a medicine that contains bismuth, such as Pepto-Bismol. Barium and bismuth may cause inaccurate results.
Thyroid scan and thyroid uptake	• Thyroid scan: Uses a radioactive tracer and a camera to provide information on the size, shape, and location of the gland, as well as the gland's overall activity. • Thyroid uptake: Measures thyroid function but does not involve imaging.	• Thyroid scan: Radioactive iodine is administered in liquid or tablet form. If iodine is given in tablet form, the patient will come back for the scan in 4 to 24 hours. If it is given by IV route, the scan may be performed within 30 minutes. • The tracer travels through the patient's body, and the camera measures how much is absorbed by the thyroid. A thyroid scan takes about 30 minutes. The patient must lie down and remain still for the procedure. • For a thyroid uptake, the patient sits in a chair for the approximately 30-minute procedure. • Within hours or a few days following the administration of radioactive iodine, the tracer is passed in urine and stool.	Seafood and iodine-rich foods should be avoided for 3 days prior to the exam. As well, CT and angiography should be avoided for 1 week prior to the exam, and thyroid replacement or suppressive therapy discontinued 1 week before the exam.
ECG/EKG (electrocardiography) *For a sample requisition, see Appendix 7.5: ECG/EKG Requisition.*	• Measures the heart's electrical activity to determine whether it is normal or irregular, and thus determine functioning. • May be recommended if a patient is experiencing arrhythmia, chest pain, or palpitations.	• An ECG (sometimes called an EKG) is a painless, non-invasive procedure. A number of electrodes are attached to the patient's chest, arm, and leg by small adhesive patches. • The patient lies still during the test, which usually takes 5–10 minutes.	None required.

X-RAY

Images are produced on special film when radiation is passed through a particular part of the body.

For a sample requisition, see Appendix 7.6: General X-Ray Requisition.

Imaging Technique	About the Test	What to Expect	Preparation
Bone densitometry	Uses a very low-dose X-ray to determine whether the patient has osteoporosis by measuring how many grams of calcium and other minerals are present in a segment of bone.	• Machines differ depending on the body part being scanned. The patient may lie down on a table for a hip or spine scan, or a portable device may be used to image a foot or forearm. • While the picture is being taken, the patient must hold still and may be asked to briefly hold his or her breath.	• None required.
Mammography *For a sample requisition, see Appendix 7.7: Mammography Requisition.*	Uses a low-dose X-ray for either screening for or diagnosis of breast disease.	• The breast tissue is gently but firmly compressed by the mammography unit. The compression allows the radiation dose to be kept to a minimum and helps distinguish breast tissue. The compression may be uncomfortable, but does not last for very long.	• None required.
Lower GI tract (colonoscopy and sigmoidoscopy)	Uses an X-ray to image the lower intestine (colon), sigmoid colon, and rectum in order to detect polyps, cancer, or ulcerative colitis.	• The patient lies on his or her back on the examination table and a probe is placed in the rectum. The probe releases a mixture of water and barium, which travels either to the sigmoid colon or all the way through the large colon, depending on the test; air is inserted to help widen the colon. • The table will be positioned at different angles and a series of X-rays taken to view the colon or sigmoid colon. • The patient must keep still and may be asked to briefly hold his or her breath while each X-ray is taken. • During the procedure, the patient may feel pressure and may worry that he or she will empty the bowel. As soon as the procedure is complete, the patient will be assisted to the washroom, where the barium and air are expelled. • The patient may return to a normal diet but is encouraged to drink plenty of water for the next 24 hours. The first bowel movements after the procedure will produce white stool.	• The colon must be completely empty for the procedure. For the day before the procedure, the patient will be asked to follow a diet of clear liquids and to use a laxative or enema (specific instructions will be given by the physician). • Cleansing of the colon is more important for the colonoscopy, as it looks at the rectum, sigmoid colon, and large intestine, while the sigmoidoscopy views only the rectum and sigmoid colon. • For a colonoscopy, the patient will be given an anesthetic and other medications to keep him or her drowsy and relaxed before this procedure. A sigmoidoscopy does not require medication, but patients who are anxious about the test can discuss taking something to help relieve the anxiety with their physician.
Upper GI tract	Uses an X-ray to examine the stomach, esophagus, and duodenum to detect ulcers, tumours, blockages, and **hiatal hernias**.	• The radiologist will watch the barium (see the Preparation column) pass down the patient's esophagus into the stomach using a **fluoroscope**. • The patient will be placed on an exam table, which will be positioned at different angles. Some positions may be uncomfortable, but each will not last very long. Once the digestive tract is covered in barium, X-rays are taken. • The examination may cause a feeling of bloating. Stools over the next 24 hours may be white or grey.	• The patient will drink liquid barium, which has a chalky flavour and may seem thick and difficult to swallow.

ULTRASONOGRAPHY (ULTRASOUND)

A non-invasive procedure that uses sound waves to assess body structures; most commonly used for abdominal, pelvic, and obstetrical evaluation.

For a sample requisition, see Appendix 7.8: Ultrasound Requisition.

Imaging Technique	About the Test	What to Expect	Preparation
Pelvic	Used to examine the reproductive organs and bladder.	• The patient will lie down, and an ultrasound technologist will apply gel to the skin over the area to be scanned (the abdomen, for example), then place an ultrasound transducer on the skin. The results are processed by the ultrasound computer into detailed images. • The procedure uses no **ionizing radiation**.	• A full bladder is required to properly visualize the pelvic organs and structures. • Ninety minutes before the exam, the patient should empty his or her bladder and drink one litre of water over a 30-minute period. • The patient should not empty the bladder until instructed to do so by the technologist, when the examination is complete.
Transvaginal	Used to look at a woman's reproductive organs, including the uterus, ovaries, and cervix, to discover whether she has cysts, fibroid tumours, or other growths; infertility; or ectopic pregnancy.	• The patient lies down on a table with knees bent. A probe (transducer) covered with a condom and lubricant gel is inserted into the vagina, and the doctor or ultrasound technician views pictures of the pelvic organs on a monitor. • The test is usually painless, but the pressure of the probe may cause some discomfort.	• The patient must empty her bladder before the procedure.
Abdominal	Used to examine the kidneys, liver, gallbladder, pancreas, spleen, and the abdominal aorta.	• (Same as Pelvic, above.)	Preparation depends on the area of study: • Liver, gallbladder, spleen, and pancreas testing may require a fat-free meal on the evening before the test and then fasting for 8 to 12 hours before the test. • Kidneys: The patient will need to drink 6 to 12 glasses of liquid an hour before the test, and may be asked to fast for 8 to 12 hours before the test to avoid extra gas in the intestines. • Aorta: The patient may need to fast for 8 to 12 hours before the test.
Obstetrical	Used to examine the fetus and cervix.	• (Same as Pelvic, above.)	• A full bladder is required to properly visualize the fetus if pregnancy is in the early stages. • The patient may be required to empty her bladder 40 to 90 minutes before the exam and then drink one litre of water within a 30-minute period and hold it until after the procedure is performed.
Breast imaging *For a sample requisition, see Appendix 7.7 Mammography Requisition.*	Most often used for assessment of a mammographic finding to determine whether it is solid or **cystic**. Breast ultrasonography is also used to evaluate palpable lumps not seen with mammography and in very dense breast tissue.	• (Same as Pelvic, above.)	• None required.

CT SCAN

A safe, noninvasive test that uses X-ray and computer technology to produce cross-sectional images of different parts of the body.

For a sample requisition, see Appendix 7.9: CT Requisition.

Imaging Technique	About the Test	What to Expect	Preparation
CT scan (general)	CT images provide greater detail than X-ray images and a more accurate assessment of organs. They are often administered when abnormalities are found on other tests, such as X-rays or ultrasounds.	• Typically, contrast material (a dye that enhances the contrast of structures or fluids within the body) is used to aid in viewing internal organs, arteries and veins, soft tissues, brain, breasts, and the digestive tract. It is not used when viewing bones. • If contrast is required, it will be delivered in IV, drink, or enema form. • Contrast material commonly causes a warm/flush sensation in the body and/or a metallic taste in the mouth. • The patient lies on a narrow table that slides into CT scanner, and X-ray beams rotate around him or her. The patient must lie very still and may be asked to hold his or her breath for short periods of time. The scan takes a few minutes.	• Most CT exams do not require any special preparation; however, the patient may be asked not to eat or drink for a few hours beforehand. • The radiologist should be aware of all the patient's medications and allergies (if any), and of any other medical conditions, especially heart disease, asthma, diabetes, kidney disease, or thyroid problems, as these may increase the risk of adverse reaction to the contrast material.
Total body scan	This diagnostic CT, which has become popular in recent years, provides very high-quality and detailed pictures of the body organs and tissues. The imaging concentrates on the chest and abdomen, and can detect subtle abnormalities of the lungs and abdominal organs.	• Same as procedure outlined above, but does not require contrast dye.	• None required.
Virtual colonoscopy/ Colonography CT	A test that allows viewing of the inside of the colon without the invasive procedure described above.	• A small tube is inserted into the rectum to inflate the colon. This is to straighten the colon as much as possible so that polyps or other growths are not hidden in its folds. The table then moves through the scanner, with the patient on his or her back. The patient may be asked to hold his or her breath for 15 seconds. Then, the patient flips onto his or her stomach and the procedure is repeated. • The entire exam takes about 15 minutes.	• Preparation is similar to that of a colonoscopy: bowel-emptying diet and laxatives. Details of how to cleanse the bowels are given by the testing centre.

TABLE 7.2 Common Office Tests

Test	Description and Preparation	
Urinalysis	Testing urine provides information about a person's health. It may identify possible reasons for certain symptoms (e.g., excessive thirst, painful urination) or reveal diseases that do not have overt signs or symptoms (e.g., diabetes, glomerulonephritis). Urine is collected in a specimen container. The office administrator will dip a chemstrip (dipstick) into the urine, wait a minute, and then compare the dipped stick with pictures on the side of the bottle or, alternatively, process the chemstrip in a urine strip analyzer. (If you do not check the stick within or at one minute, you must dip a new stick for accurate results.) The bottle or strip will indicate whether the urine is abnormal. Normal urine varies from colourless to dark yellow and is clear. Abnormal urine may be cloudy (meaning there are suspended particles, such as red blood cells or crystals, in it), red to brownish in colour (may contain blood), or have a greenish tint (may contain bilirubin from the liver). An abnormal result is recorded in the patient's chart. For example, if there is a high concentration of leukocytes, the office administrator will record "leuc++"; the number of plus symbols indicates how high the number of leucocytes present is. If there are abnormalities in the patient's urine or if the patient is experiencing symptoms but the urine tests negative (normal), the urine will be sent for further testing. Collected urine must be stored in the refrigerator until it is picked up by the laboratory for microscopic analysis.	**Preparation:** No preparation is required unless a **midstream** sample is requested. To collect a midstream sample, the patient should urinate a little, wipe the area, urinate into the sterile container, remove the sterile container from the stream, and finish urinating. Example of a sterile container that may be used to collect a urine sample. Containers are obtained from a laboratory facility, such as LifeLabs or Canadian Medical Laboratories. SOURCE: Kyle Simpson / Dreamstime.com. Chemstrip Multistix SOURCE: Universal Images Group Limited / Alamy.
Pregnancy test	A **pregnancy test strip** is very economical and easy to use. This type of "dip and read" test is designed for rapid qualitative diagnosis of **hCG (human chorionic gonadotropin) pregnancy hormone** in urine. Simply dip the strip into a urine specimen and allow five minutes for development of results, which will either show a control line (indicating negative pregnancy test results) or control and test line (indicating positive pregnancy test results).	**Preparation:** None required. Note that the first morning urine will have the strongest amount of hCG hormone present.
Throat swab	A throat swab may be used to detect the presence of Group A *Streptococcus* bacteria (the most common cause of strep throat). The patient will be asked to tilt his or her head back and open the mouth wide. The health care provider, or nurse if there is one in the office, will rub a sterile cotton swab along the back of the patient's throat near the tonsils. The swab is sealed and sent to a lab for diagnosis. The patient may feel a gagging sensation when the swab is placed at the back of the throat.	**Preparation:** None required. Throat Swab SOURCE: Maria DeCambra. Used with permission.

Test	Description and Preparation	
Papanicolaou (Pap) test	A Pap test checks for changes in the cells of the cervix. The Pap test can tell if the patient has an infection, abnormal (unhealthy) cervical cells, or cervical cancer. Getting regular Pap tests is important to prevent cervical cancer and screen for other diseases. The patient lies on a table with her feet in stirrups. The doctor or nurse places an instrument called a speculum into the vagina and opens it slightly; this allows the doctor or nurse to better see inside the vagina and cervix. Cells are gently scraped from the cervix area and sent to a lab for examination. Two samples are usually taken—one of mucus from the cervix and one of tissue. The Pap slide containing the smear is sent to the lab for evaluation. (For a sample requisition, see Appendix 7.10: Pap Test Requisition.) The doctor or nurse should be aware of all medications the patient is taking; some birth control pills that contain estrogen or progestin may interfere with test results. Pap tests should not be scheduled when the patient is menstruating, as this may affect the accuracy of the test.	**Preparation:** The patient should empty her bladder just before the test. The test may cause some discomfort, similar to menstrual cramps. Some pressure may also be felt during the test, and some minor bleeding may occur afterward. Pap Smear Slide and Sample Tools SOURCE: Maria DeCambra. Used with permission.
Sexually transmitted infection (STI) tests	Sexually transmitted infections (STIs) are among the most pervasive infections in the world. An STI can affect a person's general well-being and reproductive ability. It is easier to prevent an STI than to treat one once it has been contracted. Depending on the patient's symptoms, the doctor or nurse may examine the genitals and may take a swab from the urethra (in men) or vagina and/or cervix (in women), and from a lesion or sore, if present. The patient may also be asked to give a urine sample and/or take a blood test. See Appendix 7.11: *Chlamydia* Swab Specimen Collection Instructions.	**Preparation:** The patient should not urinate during the two hours prior to the check-up. Swab for *Chlamydia* SOURCE: Maria DeCambra. Used with permission.
Eye exam	An eye exam in the doctor's office involves an eye chart and relevant history. The physician will also test the eye using an ophthalmoscope to examine inside the eye, including the retina and the optic nerve. On the **Snellen chart**, the patient is shown 11 rows of capital letters. The top row contains one letter (usually the "big E," but other letters can be used). The other rows contain letters that are progressively smaller. For children, the eye chart may contain pictures or only the big E facing in different directions and gradually getting smaller. The standard placement of the eye chart is on a wall 20 feet away from the patient's eyes. Because many doctors' offices do not have rooms that are 20 feet long, they may or may not decide to check **visual acuity**. When checking visual acuity, the doctor covers one of the patient's eyes at a time and the vision of each eye is recorded separately, as well as both eyes together. In the Snellen fraction 20/20, the first number represents the test distance, 20 feet. The second number represents the distance that the average eye can see the letters on a certain line of the eye chart. So, 20/20 means that the eye being tested can read a certain size letter when it is 20 feet away. If a person sees 20/40—that is, at 40 feet from the chart—he or she can read letters that a person with 20/20 vision could read from 20 feet away.	**Preparation:** None required. Snellen Eye Charts for Adults and Children SOURCE: © Mpavlov / Dreamstime.com.

Test	Description and Preparation	
Stool tests	A doctor may order a stool collection to test for a variety of possible conditions, including allergy, infection (bacteria, virus, or parasites in the gastrointestinal tract), digestive problems (malabsorption of sugar or fats), and bleeding of the GI tract. Most often, blood streaking the stool is from a rectal tear (fissure) or hemorrhoids, not from an illness or disease. Stool samples may be collected as a smear on a card or in a container. See Appendix 7.12: Stool, Ova, and Parasite Specimen Instructions. The stool is sent to the laboratory to test for blood, bacteria, or ova and parasites. Swabs of the rectum may also be taken to check for viruses.	Container Sample for Stool Test 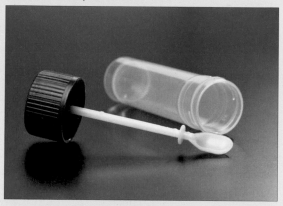 SOURCE: © Luchschen / Dreamstime.com.
Pulmonary function tests (PFTs)	Pulmonary function tests are done to test for allergies and chronic lung conditions. There are many types of PFTs; however, in the physician's office the common PFT used is spirometry. Spirometry measures lung function by measuring airflow—how much air the patient exhales, and how quickly. It can evaluate a broad range of lung disorders and diseases, such as asthma, bronchitis, and emphysema. It may also allow the doctor to discover the cause of shortness of breath or the effect of exposure to chemicals. The patient will be asked to sit down and breathe into a mouthpiece that fits tightly over the mouth. The patient must breathe through the mouth, not the nose. He or she will take in a big breath and then force it out as hard and long as possible into the mouthpiece. This procedure may be repeated three times or more. The mouthpiece is connected to an instrument called a spirometer. The PFT provides information on lung volume, capacity, rate of flow, and gas exchange. The patient may also be asked to inhale a substance or a medicine and then repeat the test. This will allow the physician to see the effect on the test results. For example, if the physician suspects asthma, the patient may be asked to try a bronchodilator and repeat the test to see whether the medication improved the patient's performance.	**Preparation:** Patients should not eat a heavy meal, smoke for 4 to 6 hours, or drink alcohol one hour before the test. Patients using bronchodilators or inhaler medications will receive specific instructions if they are required to stop using these prior to the test. Because spirometry involves some forced and rapid breathing, patients may experience temporary shortness of breath or lightheadedness following the test. Spirometer 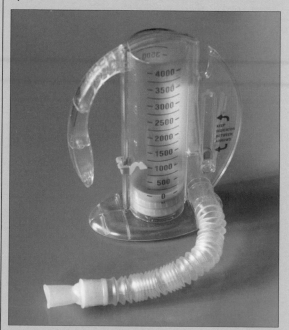 SOURCE: © Susanne Neal / Dreamstime.com.

Test	Description and Preparation
Weight and height	Taking a patient's weight at the doctor's office is standard procedure for an annual health exam and well-baby check. There are health risks associated with both underweight and overweight individuals: Underweight: • undernutrition (or eating disorder) • osteoporosis • infertility • impaired immunocompetence Overweight: • type 2 diabetes • dyslipidemia • hypertension • coronary heart disease, gallbladder disease • obstructive sleep apnea • certain cancers Body mass index (BMI) and waist circumference (WC) are two commonly used methods to gauge an individual's health risk. Waist circumference is also an important indicator of vulnerability for certain health risks, such as high blood pressure, heart disease, stroke, high blood cholesterol, and type 2 diabetes. The BMI is a number calculated by correlating a person's weight and height, and is used to demonstrate which weight category an individual falls under. Any weight category outside of normal may lead to health problems. BMI indexing is used only on adults aged 20 and older. <table><tr><th>Category</th><th>BMI Range (kg/m^2)</th></tr><tr><td>Very severely underweight</td><td>less than 15</td></tr><tr><td>Severely underweight</td><td>from 15 to 16</td></tr><tr><td>Underweight</td><td>from 16 to 18.5</td></tr><tr><td>Normal (healthy weight)</td><td>from 18.5 to 25</td></tr><tr><td>Overweight</td><td>from 25 to 30</td></tr><tr><td>Obese Class I (Moderately obese)</td><td>from 30 to 35</td></tr><tr><td>Obese Class II (Severely obese)</td><td>from 35 to 40</td></tr><tr><td>Obese Class III (Very severely obese)</td><td>over 40</td></tr></table> Sex-specific cut-off points for WC (demonstrating extent of excessive abdominal fat) have been established to identify whether an individual is at risk for certain diseases, one of which is metabolic syndrome (considered a risk factor for cardiovascular diseases and type 2 diabetes). For men: WC ≥ 102 cm (40 in) For women: WC ≥ 88 cm (35 in) See Appendix 7.13: Weight and Height Charts for Adults and Children.

RESOURCES

Canadian Institute for Health Information:
http://www.cihi.ca/CIHI-ext-portal/internet/en/tabbedcontent/types+of+care/specialized+services/medical+imaging/cihi010642

Canadian Medical Association point-of-care tools:
http://cma.ca/pointofcare?WT.mc_id=AW1301395&WT.srch=1 (Note: You must be a member of the CMA to use most of these tools.)

Ontario Ministry of Health Central Repository for Laboratory Services: http://www.forms.ssb.gov.on.ca/mbs/ssb/forms/ssbforms.nsf/FormDetail?OpenForm&ACT=RDR&TAB=PROFILE&SRCH=&ENV=WWE&TIT=4471&NO=014-4471-44E

Ontario Ministry of Health for Health Professionals:
http://www.health.gov.on.ca/en/pro/

Links to Original Forms

CML Health Care:
http://cmlhealthcare.com/healthcare-provider/

CT Scan:
http://www.kgh.on.ca/en/specialtiesandservices/Imaging Services/Documents/CT_Requisition.pdf

Cytology Requisition (including Pap):
http://www.gamma-dynacare.ca/Files/Content/Cytology Requisition - Ontario %5BPDF%5D.pdf

Gamma Dynacare Medical Laboratories:
http://www.gamma-dynacare.ca/Content/HealthcareProviders/DownloadableForms.aspx?expandable=1

Histopathology Requisition:
http://www.gamma-dynacare.ca/Files/Content/Histology Requisition - Ontario %5BPDF%5D.pdf

Imaging Requisition:
http://www.kgh.on.ca/en/specialtiesandservices/Imaging Services/Documents/Imaging Requisition.pdf

Laboratory Requisitions:
http://www.forms.ssb.gov.on.ca/mbs/ssb/forms/ssbforms.nsf/GetFileAttach/014-4422-84~1/$File/4422-84.pdf

LifeLabs Medical Laboratory Services:
http://www.lifelabs.com/Lifelabs_ON/Health_Care/Specimen-Handling-and-Collection-Instructions.asp

Mammography:
http://www.kgh.on.ca/en/healthcareprofessionals/Documents/Breast Assessment Requisition.pdf

MRI:
http://www.kgh.on.ca/en/specialtiesandservices/Imaging Services/Documents/KGH MRI Requisition Aug 2013.pdf

REVIEW QUESTIONS

True or False?

1. The office administrator may file test results if they are received with all values in the optimal range.
2. Females between the ages of 21 and 65 must have a Pap test every year.
3. Waist circumference may be an indicator of health risk.
4. The four key categories for imaging are CT, nuclear medicine, radiography, and blood work.
5. Urine specimens must be kept in the fridge until they are delivered to the lab.
6. Men and women are measured equally on the BMI chart.

Fill in the Blank

1. A _____ test is administered to patients who are not showing any symptoms.
2. The following patient information—address, name, phone number, health card number—are all part of the _____ of a patient requisition.
3. Blood and _____ tests are the most common screening and diagnostic tests.
4. A(n) _____ provides detailed, cross-sectional images of body organs and tissues using a magnetic field and radio waves passing through the body.
5. Thyroid uptake measures _____ function and requires the patient to sit in a chair for approximately _____.
6. Pelvic ultrasonography is used to examine the _____ and the bladder.
7. A CBC counts the number of red blood cells, the different types of white blood cells, and platelets in the blood. It also measures _____ and _____ levels.
8. A Pap test checks for changes in the cells of the _____.

Multiple Choice

1. A patient's weight is important. If a patient is underweight, the physician may be concerned about all but ONE of the following:

    a. infertility

    b. osteoporosis

    c. hypertension

    d. eating disorder

2. Two common methods used to gauge the effect of patients' weight on their health are

    a. waist circumference and weight

    b. weight and body mass index

    c. weight and height

    d. waist circumference and body mass index

3. A PFT measures

    a. lung function

    b. airway obstruction

    c. nasal congestion

    d. heart rate

4. Which one of the following tests is NOT completed by a GP?

    a. urinalysis

    b. weight

    c. Pap test

    d. blood work

5. An upper and lower GI examines the

    a. genitourinary tract

    b. gastrointestinal tract

    c. urinary tract

    d. digestive tract

6. The most common site that a phlebotomist uses to draw blood is the

    a. heel

    b. skull

    c. elbow

    d. neck

Short Answer

1. Explain why blood tests are the most common test requested by the family physician.

2. Briefly describe the path of test results received, from receipt to placement in the chart.

3. What is the Snellen fraction? How does it work?

4. PTT and INR blood test results are often received verbally. Why?

5. Explain the difference between screening and diagnostic tests.

6. Define BMI and explain what it is used for.

7. What waist circumference, for a man and for a woman, indicates that the patient may be at metabolic risk?

8. What is nuclear medicine imaging used for? Explain the imaging technology used and the required preparation(s).

HYBRID LEARNING

1. Choose two of the imaging techniques described in this chapter, and provide a detailed description of each in paragraph form. Each answer should be approximately 100–150 words. List the sources you used.

2. Do you feel that the BMI chart is an accurate measure of obesity? Find one article that suggests the BMI chart is an accurate measure and one that disputes this form of measurement. Summarize each argument in 100–150 words.

3. Obesity rates are much more common in Canadian society today than they were at any time in the past. Search for the CBC News article "Canada's obesity rates triple in less than 30 years." Watch the news report and provide a 200-word summary.

ACTIVITIES

1. You arrive at the office and find today's incoming lab reports. Your task is to process them. Consider the following:

   a. What is the first step you will take when receiving lab reports?

   b. Which lab reports do you present to the physician? Explain.

   c. When will the lab reports be ready to file?

   d. What do you expect when the lab reports are returned to you? Will they be ready for filing, or will you have to complete any tasks? Explain.

2. Search for the video titled "Mammogram Visit" on the BC Cancer Screening YouTube channel. Watch the video, which provides an overview of the procedure for a mammography. List the steps that a patient goes through when completing this test. What does the video suggest a patient can do to help make the procedure more comfortable?

3. Requisitions must be filled in correctly to ensure accurate and prompt test results. Review the following two patient cases. Then, choose the appropriate requisitions from the appendices in this chapter, and fill them out with the patient information provided.

   a. Mary Horton went to her GP complaining of a wet cough, wheezing, and chest pain. After the examination, the physician believes that Mary has pneumonia in her left lung. He writes a prescription for clindamycin HCl oral 450 mg every 6 to 8 hours. The doctor would like a follow-up appointment with Mary in four or five days, and requests that you fill in requisitions for a chest X-ray of the left lung, CBC, and differential.

   Patient information:

   Mary Horton

   Weight: 60 kg

   Address: 58 Woods Rd., Kingston, ON K7M 3T4

   DOB: Aug. 10, 1959

   HC# 6123456891 GY

   Phone: 613-544-9152

   Physician information:

   Dr. J. Gutels

   Address: 6211 Eagle St., Kingston, ON K7L 5A6

   Contact no. 613-452-5896

   Practitioner no. 258914

   b. Gary Haynes went to his GP complaining of a burning pain and stiffness in the big toe of his right foot. After examination, the physician believes that Gary has gout in his right big toe. The doctor writes a prescription for colchicine 1.2 mg for the first dose, to be followed by 0.6 mg one hour later. Further recommendations include resting the affected joint and using ice to reduce swelling. The physician requests that you fill in requisitions to include an X-ray and a blood uric acid test.

   Patient information:

   Gary Haynes

   Weight: 95 kg

   Address: 621 Albert Ave., Kingston, ON K7P 3T2

   DOB: September 11, 1949

   HC# 2154879245 YX

   Phone: 613-548-3541

   Physician information:

   Dr. J. Gutels

   Address: 6211 Eagle St., Kingston, ON K7L 5A6

   Contact no. 613-452-5896

   Practitioner no. 258914

4. Refer to the BMI chart in Appendix 7.13. Indicate both the BMI value and the category under which each patient falls. (Use the conversion chart in Appendix 7.19 to convert height in centimetres to inches and weight from kilograms to pounds, rounding figures up or down.)

   a. 152 cm and 45 kg   **e.** 183 cm and 113 kg

   b. 168 cm and 90 kg   **f.** 147 cm and 112 kg

   c. 188 cm and 92 kg   **g.** 193 cm and 109 kg

   d. 175 cm and 160 kg   **h.** 157 cm and 59 kg

5. Refer to the optimal range for blood test results in Appendix 7.19. Indicate whether the following results are considered optimal or non-optimal.

	Female	Male
Glucose	98	80
Cholesterol	185	210
Low-density lipoprotien (LDL)	105	110
High-density lipoprotien (HDL)	52	62
Triglycerides	98	85
WBC	7.8	9.2
RBC	3	4.3
Hemoglobin	13.2	14
OGTT 2 h	13.2	6.8

6. The following patients were in to see the physician today. All of them need requisitions completed for further testing. Please complete the correct requisition(s) for each patient. You are working for Dr. J. Gutels, 6211 Eagle St., Kingston, ON K7L 5A6; contact no. 613-452-5896, practitioner no. 258914. Use the requisition links provided in the resources at the end of the chapter.

Encounter	Patient Information
a. Amell was in today complaining of a sore R knee joint. When the joint is manipulated, there is a fair amount of pain. I have prescribed Celebrex 100 mg bid x 2 rpts to help reduce inflammation and sent for X-ray. Please fill in imaging requisition and give to patient. R/c 2/52 to discuss results of X-ray.	Amell Danita DOB: 1949-03-15 345 Stuart St. Kingston, ON K8R 5J6 Phone: 613-542-8946 HC# 4444444444 XY
b. Michelle was in today complaining of frequent headaches. Headaches are severe enough to cause vomiting. Very photosensitive. I believe patient is suffering from migraines. Have ordered CT scan to R/O other causes. Prescribed Axert 12.5 mg 1 PO OD. Mitte: 30. R/c 1/12.	Michelle Kendall DOB: 1989-03-26 1073 Maclean St. Kingston, ON K7K 1S6 Phone: 613-431-6568 HC# 7639280002
c. Gilbert was in today. Patient was in a car accident 1 week ago and T3–T7 on L side extremely tender. Am sending for chest X-ray to rule out cracked ribs.	Gilbert Trinidad DOB: 1949-06-15 22 South St. Kingston, ON K7M3X3 Phone: 613-344-5566 HC# 4521780215 VC
d. Chung was in today for minor surgery on her nose. She has an irregular, dark brown lesion on nose that was first noted 2 months ago and has increased in size to approx. 2 mm x 3 mm. Small growth was removed and needs to be sent to lab. Sample was excised at 11:15 a.m. today.	Chung Choi DOB: 1933-07-10 5 Gardiners Rd. Kingston, ON K7M 2A1 Phone: 613-532-6396 HC# 8321785431
e. Hassan was in today for a general annual exam. Would like the following blood work completed: CBC, lipid assessment, random glucose.	Hassan Hamalah DOB: 1955-05-17 1959 Forest Valley Dr. Kingston, ON K7K 1W1 Phone: 613-431-8599 HC# 1984685964 AX
f. Jade was in at 2:00 p.m. today for a routine Pap. Her LMP was June 20, 2014. Took cervical smear with spatula. She is on Alesse. She was not vaccinated for HPV. Please fill in req. and send with smear.	Jade Boersma DOB: 1961-10-09 68 Deerway Lane Kingston, ON K2K 5H3 Phone: 613-685-4595 HC# 8624996347 GH

APPENDIX 7.11

Chlamydia Swab Specimen Collection Instructions

Chlamydia/Neisseria gonorrhoeae (GC) Swab Specimen Collection

1. Open GenProbe Aptima Collection kit.
   DO NOT TOUCH TOP OF CAP on the collection tube.

2. Remove excess mucus from cervical os using cleaning WHITE shaft swab. DISCARD this swab.

3. Insert specimen collection BLUE shaft swab into endocervical canal. Rotate swab clockwise for 10 to 30 seconds.

4. Remove cap from swab transport tube (DO NOT TOUCH TOP OF CAP) and place swab into transport tube.

5. Break swab shaft at the scoreline. Re-cap tube tightly. DO NOT TOUCH TOP OF FOIL CAP.

6. Ensure sample is properly labelled with patient's full name, plus one other identifier (e.g., DOB). If using adhesive label, labels should be small enough to fit ENTIRELY on the tube to prevent tearing off in the sample rack.

7. Place collection tube/specimen into individual zip lock bag to prevent cross-contamination. 1 PATIENT SPECIMEN PER BAG.

8. Remove gloves carefully, wash hands immediately.

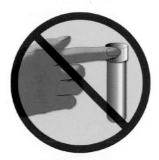

DO NOT TOUCH TOP OF FOIL CAP

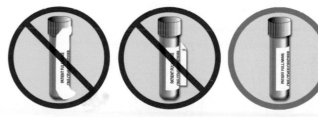

LABELS SHOULD FIT ENTIRELY ON SAMPLE TUBE

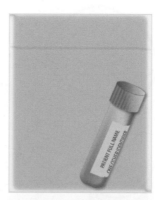

1 PATIENT SPECIMEN PER BAG

SOURCE: Gamma-Dynacare. Used with permission.

APPENDIX 7.12

Stool, Ova, and Parasite Specimen Instructions

LifeLabs Medical Laboratory Services
COLLECTING STOOL SAMPLES FOR MICROBIOLOGY
Patient Instructions

You have been provided one or more of the following containers:
- Stool Culture Transport Medium, Cary Blair (Pink Liquid)
- Fixative SAF, Stool Transport Medium for Ova and Parasites (Clear Liquid)
- Clean Vial (No Liquid)

Do not discard liquid.
Fill all containers provided.

1 Urinate into the toilet if needed.

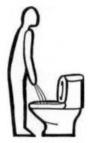

2 Lift toilet seat. Place sheets of plastic wrap (e.g., Saran Wrap) over the toilet bowl, leaving a slight dip in the centre. Place the toilet seat down. Pass stool onto plastic wrap.

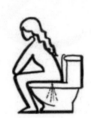

PLASTIC

3 Alternatively, use a clean bowl or sterilized bedpan. Do not let urine or water touch the stool specimen.

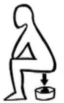

OR

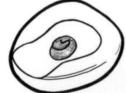

4 Using the spoon attached to the cap, place bloody or slimy/white (mucus) areas of the stool (if present) into container(s). Do not over-fill the container(s).

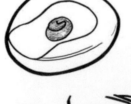

FILL LINE

5 In container(s) with liquid: Add 2–3 spoonfuls of stool until the liquid reaches the "FILL LINE." Tighten cap(s). In the empty CLEAN container (if provided): Add stool to the "FILL LINE" and tighten cap.

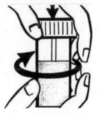

6 Shake the container(s) with liquid to mix the contents.

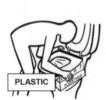

7 Wash hands with soap and water. Write Name, Date of Birth or Health Card No. and Date and Time of collection on each container. Place container(s) into plastic bag(s) and seal.

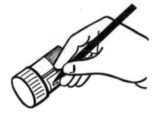

8 Bring the container(s) back to the lab within 24 hours of collection. Delays may affect test results. Until specimens can be brought to the lab, store as follows:
- CULTURE (pink liquid)—refrigerate
- SAF (clear liquid)—room temperature
- CLEAN (no liquid)—refrigerate

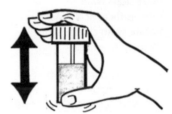

LifeLabs
Medical Laboratory Services

APPENDIX 7.13

Weight and Height Charts for Adults and Children

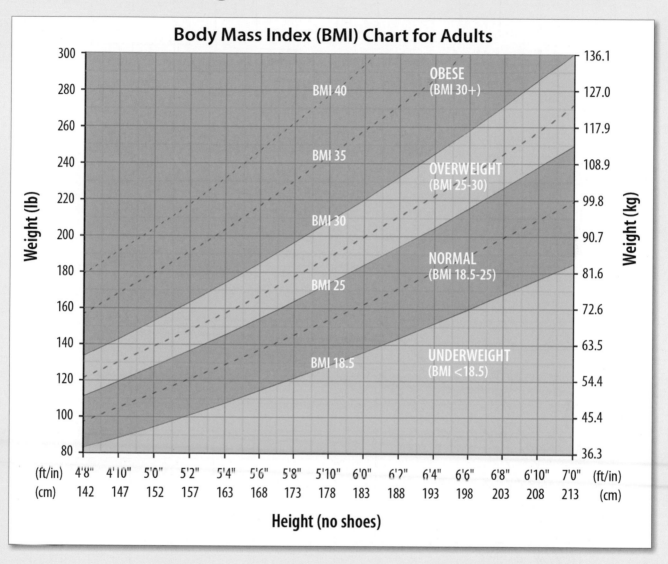

Boys' Growth Percentiles, Birth to 36 Months

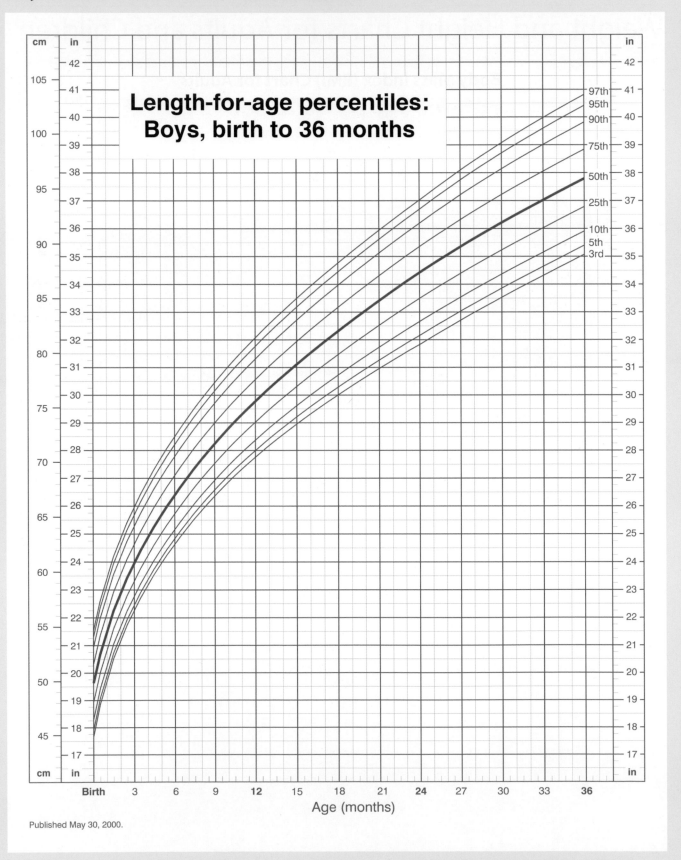

Length-for-age percentiles: Boys, birth to 36 months

Published May 30, 2000.

SOURCE: Developed by the National Center for Health Statistics in collaboration with the National Center for Chronic Disease Prevention and Health Promotion (2000).

Girls' Growth Percentiles, Birth to 36 Months

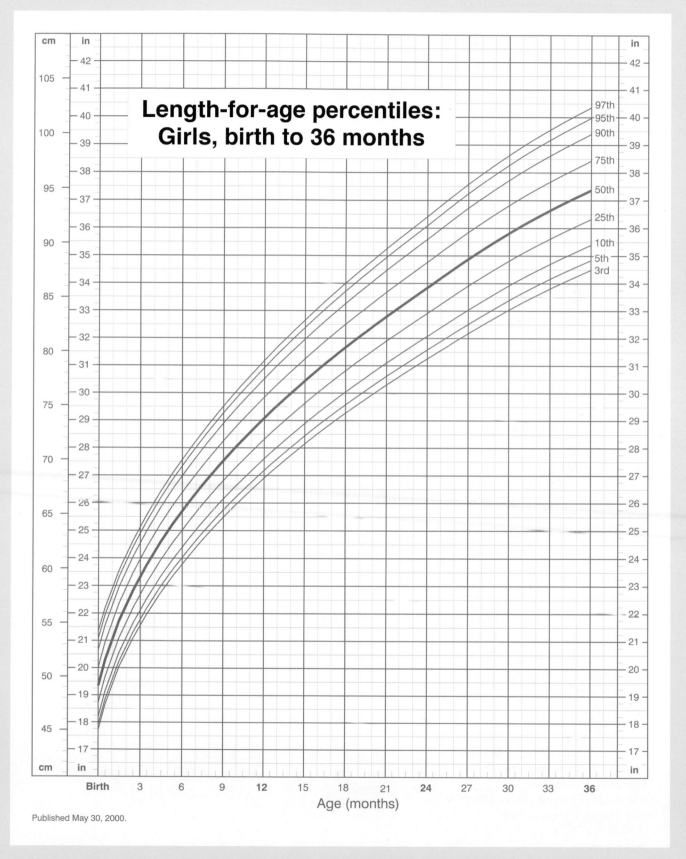

Length-for-age percentiles:
Girls, birth to 36 months

Published May 30, 2000.

SOURCE: Developed by the National Center for Health Statistics in collaboration with the National Center for Chronic Disease Prevention and Health Promotion (2000).

APPENDIX 7.14

Optimal Ranges for Common Blood Tests

The chemistry panel and complete blood count (CBC) blood tests provide a comprehensive metabolic evaluation of a patient and include the following tests:

- Fasting glucose (blood sugar)
- Uric acid
- Blood urea nitrogen (BUN): Measures liver and kidney function
- Creatinine: Measures kidney function
- BUN–creatinine ratio: For diagnosis of impaired renal function
- Estimated glomerular filtration rate (eGFR)
- Sodium
- Potassium
- Chloride
- Calcium
- Phosphorus
- Total protein
- Albumin
- Globulin
- Albumin–globulin ratio
- Bilirubin: Evaluates kidney and liver function
- Alkaline phosphatase: Evaluates liver and bone diseases
- Lactic dehydrogenase (LDH)
- AST (SGOT): Evaluates liver function
- ALT (SGPT): Evaluates liver function
- Iron (serum)
- Lipid profile: Evaluates risk for developing atherosclerosis (arterial plaque) and coronary heart disease:
  - Total cholesterol
  - Triglycerides
  - High-density lipoprotein (HDL) cholesterol
  - Low-density lipoprotein (LDL) cholesterol
  - Total cholesterol–HDL ratio
- Complete blood count (CBC):
  - Red blood cell count (RBC)
  - Hemoglobin
  - Hematocrit
  - Red blood cell indices
  - Mean corpuscular volume (MCV)
  - Mean corpuscular hemoglobin (MCH)
  - Mean corpuscular hemoglobin concentration (MCHC)
  - Red blood cell distribution width (RDW)
  - White blood cell count (WBC)
  - Differential count
  - Platelet count

Optimal ranges for common blood tests are listed in the chart below:

Test	Current Laboratory Reference Range	Optimal Range
Glucose	65–99 mg/dL	70–85 mg/dL
Cholesterol	100–199 mg/dL	180–200 mg/dL
LDL	0–99 mg/dL	Under 100 mg/dL
HDL	40–59 mg/dL	Over 55 mg/dL
Triglycerides	0–149 mg/dL	Under 100 mg/dL
CBC:		
Hemoglobin	Female: 12–16 gm/dL Male: 13–18 gm/dL	Female: 13.5–14.5 gm/dL Male: 14.0–15.0 gm/dL
Hematocrit	Female: 37–48% Male: 45–62%	Female: 37–44% Male: 40–48%
WBC	4.0–10.0 x E9/L	5.0–8.0 x E9/L
RBC	4.00–5.10 x E12/L	Female: 3.9–4.5 x E12/L Male: 4.2–4.9 x E12/L
MCV	80–100 fL	82.0–89.9 fL
MCH	27.5–33.0 pg	27.0–31.9 pg
RDW	11.5–14.5%	≤13.0%
Platelet count	150–400 x E9/L	240–400 x E9/L
Absolute		
Neutrophils	2.0–7.5 x E9/L	3.0–6.5 x E9/L
Lymphocytes	1.0–4.5 x E9/L	2.5–4.5 x E9/L
Monocytes	0.2–1.0 x E9/L	Within range
Eosinophils	0.0–0.5 x E9/L	0.0–0.3 x E9/L
Basophils	0.0–0.2 x E9/L	Within range
Ferritin/iron	Female: 35–155 µg/dL Male: 40–155 µg/dL	Female: 55–125 µg/dL Male: 55–125 µg/dL
Vitamin B12	198–615 pmol/L	400–615 pmol/L
Thyroid Stimulating Hormone (TSH)	0.5–6.0 µ units/mL	1–2 µ units/mL

Pap Test Results

<table>
<tr>
<td colspan="3">LABORATORY REPORT
FAMILY MEDICAL CENTRE   (30571)
AZ</td>
<td colspan="3"></td>
</tr>
<tr>
<td colspan="3"></td>
<td>COLLECTED DATE
03/25/03</td>
<td>RECEIVED DATE
03/27/03</td>
<td></td>
</tr>
<tr>
<td>REQUISITION NO.</td>
<td colspan="2">PHYSICIAN</td>
<td>REPORTED DATE
03/31/2003</td>
<td>OTHER I.D.</td>
<td>HOURS P.P.</td>
</tr>
<tr>
<td>PATIENT</td>
<td>DOB
04/06/1957</td>
<td>AGE
57 YRS</td>
<td>SEX
F</td>
<td>PATIENT NO.</td>
<td>ACCESSION NO.
60-BY-03-014029</td>
</tr>
<tr>
<td>REQUESTS</td>
<td>RESULTS</td>
<td>OUT OF RANGE RESULTS</td>
<td colspan="2">REFERENCE RANGE</td>
<td>UNITS</td>
</tr>
</table>

ACCESSION#: 60-BY-03-014029

<u>CYTOLOGY REPORT</u>

SPECIMEN SOURCE:
VAGINAL, CERVICAL – THINPREP

SPECIMEN ADEQUACY:
Satisfactory for evaluation.
Endocervical/transformation zone present.
No menstrual history available.

COMMENT:
Atrophic cellular pattern.

DIAGNOSIS:
NEGATIVE FOR INTRAEPITHELIAL LESION OR MALIGNANCY

This is a screening test with an inherent, but low, probability of error.
A negative report indicates a high probability of being disease free
from squamous cervical cancer and pre-cancer during the next year.

JC :JC

Verified by: Jerry CAGLE C.T. (ASCP)
(Electronic Signature on 03/31/15)

End of Report   Page: 1

APPENDIX 7.16

General Test Requisition

Public Health Ontario | Santé publique Ontario
PARTNERS FOR HEALTH | PARTENAIRES POUR LA SANTÉ

Date received	PHOL No.
yyyy / mm / dd	

General Test Requisition

ALL Sections of this Form MUST be Completed

1 - Submitter

Courier Code

Provide Return Address:

Name
Address
City & Province
Postal Code

Clinician Initial / Surname and OHIP / CPSO Number

Tel:_____   Fax:_____

cc Doctor Information

Name:_____   Tel:_____
Lab/Clinic Name:_____   Fax:_____
CPSO #:_____
Address:_____   Postal Code:_____

2 - Patient Information

Health No.		Sex	Date of Birth:
			yyyy / mm / dd
Medical Record No.			

Patient's Last Name *(per OHIP card)*   First Name *(per OHIP card)*

Patient Address

Postal Code	Patient Phone No.

Submitter Lab No.

Public Health Unit Outbreak No.

Public Health Investigator Information

Name:_____
Health Unit:_____
Tel:_____   Fax:_____

3 - Test(s) Requested *(Please see descriptions on reverse)*

Test: Enter test descriptions below

_____
_____
_____
_____
_____

Hepatitis Serology

Reason for test (Check (✓) only one box):

☐ Immune status
☐ Acute infection
☐ Chronic infection

Indicate specific viruses (Check (✓) all that apply):

☐ Hepatitis A
☐ Hepatitis B
☐ Hepatitis C *(testing only available for acute or chronic infection; no test for determining immunity to HCV is currently available)*

4 - Specimen Type and Site

☐ blood / serum   ☐ faeces   ☐ nasopharyngeal
☐ sputum   ☐ urine   ☐ vaginal smear
☐ urethral   ☐ cervix   ☐ BAL
☐ other - *(specify)*

Patient Setting

☐ physician office/clinic   ☐ ER (not admitted)
☐ inpatient (ward)   ☐ inpatient (ICU)   ☐ institution

5 - Reason for Test

☐ diagnostic   ☐ immune status
☐ needle stick   ☐ follow-up
☐ prenatal   ☐ chronic condition
☐ immunocompromised
☐ post-mortem
☐ other - *(specify)* _____

Date Collected:
yyyy / mm / dd

Onset Date:
yyyy / mm / dd

Clinical Information

☐ fever   ☐ gastroenteritis   ☐ respiratory symptoms
☐ STI   ☐ headache / stiff neck   ☐ vesicular rash
☐ pregnant   ☐ encephalitis / meningitis   ☐ maculopapular rash
☐ jaundice
☐ other - *(specify)*_____

☐ influenza high risk - *(specify)*_____
☐ recent travel - *(specify location)*_____

For HIV, please use the HIV serology form. - For referred cultures, please use the reference bacteriology form. To re-order this test requisition contact your local Public Health Laboratory and ask for form number F-SD-SCG-1000. Current version of Public Health Laboratory requisitions are available at www.publichealthontario.ca/requisitions
The personal health information is collected under the authority of the Personal Health Information Protection Act, s.36 (1)(c)(iii) for the purpose of clinical laboratory testing. If you have questions about the collection of this personal health information please contact the PHOL Manager of Customer Service at 416-235-6556 or toll free 1-877-604-4567. F-SD-SCG-1000 (08/2013)

▷ Ontario
Agency for Health Protection and Promotion
Agence de protection et de promotion de la santé

SOURCE: Reprinted with the permission of Public Health Ontario. © 2015 Ontario Agency for Health Protection and Promotion. The general test requisition form pictured here is an example only and subject to change. For an up-to-date general test requisition form from Public Health Ontario, please visit http://www.publichealthontario.ca/en/eRepository/General_test_fillable_requisition.pdf.

APPENDIX 7.17

Microbiology Requisition

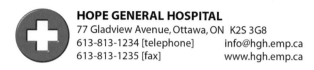

HOPE GENERAL HOSPITAL
77 Gladview Avenue, Ottawa, ON K2S 3G8
613-813-1234 [telephone]   info@hgh.emp.ca
613-813-1235 [fax]   www.hgh.emp.ca

MICROBIOLOGY REQUISITION

Date	Patient Name	
Time	Street Address	
Requesting Physician	City and Province	
Signature	Postal Code	
Diagnosis and Reason for Test	Home Phone	Alternate Phone
	Date of Birth (yyyy-mm-dd)	Sex: M☐ F☐
	List Antibiotics Currently in Use	

Specimen Type		Tests Requested
Fluids	**Respiratory**	☐ Routine Bacteriology
☐ Blood	☐ Bronchial Wash	☐ Anaerobic Culture
☐ CSF	☐ BAL	☐ Fungus Culture
☐ Joint Fluid	☐ Sputum-Expectoration	☐ Mycobacteria (TB)
☐ Pleural Fluid	☐ Trach Aspirate	☐ Group B Strep Screen
☐ CAPD Dialysate	☐ Nose	☐ Genital Mycoplasma
☐ Other	☐ Throat	☐ *C. difficile* Toxin
Others	**Urine**	☐ MRSA Screen
☐ Vagina	☐ Midstream	☐ VRE Screen
☐ Cervix	☐ Cysto	☐ Gonorrhea
☐ Urethra	☐ Indwelling Catheter	☐ *Chlamydia trachomatis*
☐ Eye: ☐Right ☐Left	☐ In/Out Catheter	☐ Legionella
☐ Ear: ☐Right ☐Left	☐ Other:	☐ PCP
☐ Stools	**Dialysis**	☐ Other
☐ Wound	☐ **Water** ☐ **Pre** ☐ **Post**	**Additional Information:**
☐ Other:	☐ **Dialysate** ☐ **Pre** ☐ **Post**	
CC Physician		

APPENDIX 7.18

Laboratory Requisition

HOPE GENERAL HOSPITAL
77 Gladview Avenue, Ottawa, ON K2S 3G8
613-813-1234 [telephone]   info@hgh.emp.ca
613-813-1235 [fax]   www.hgh.emp.ca

[If in a setting that has an addressograph, imprint patient information here.]

LABORATORY REQUISITION

Please bring your requisition and OHIP card to your appointment. Arrive at least 15 minutes prior to scheduled appointment.

Requisitioning Practitioner	Address
Facility No. / CPSO No.	Clinician/Practitioner's Contact Number for Urgent Results

Name (as it appears on Health Card)

Sex ☐ M ☐ F Date of Birth (yyyy mm dd)	Service Date
Address	Postal Code
Home Phone	Work Phone	Cell Phone

Check One   ☐ OHIP/Insured   ☐ Third Party/Uninsured   ☐ WSIB

Health Card Number (OHIP)   Version Code (if applicable)

Card Expiry Date (if applicable)

BIOCHEMISTRY	HEMATOLOGY	Viral Hepatitis (check one only)
☐ Glucose ☐ Random ☐ Fasting	☐ CBC	☐ Acute Hepatitis
☐ HbA1C	☐ Prothrombin Time (INR)	☐ Chronic Hepatitis
☐ TSH	**IMMUNOLOGY**	☐ Immune Status/Previous Exposure
☐ Creatinine (eGFR)	☐ Pregnancy test (Urine)	Specify ☐ Hepatitis A
☐ Uric Acid	☐ Mononucleosis Screen	☐ Hepatitis B
☐ Sodium	☐ Rubella	☐ Hepatitis C
☐ Potassium	☐ Prenatal: ABO, RhD, Antibody Screen (titre and ident. If positive)	Or order individual hepatitis tests in the "Other Tests" section below
☐ Chloride		
☐ CK	☐ Repeat Prenatal Antibodies	
☐ ALT	**Microbiology ID & Sensitivities (if warranted)**	**Prostate Specific Antigen (PSA)**
☐ Alk. Phosphate	☐ Cervical	☐ Total PSA ☐ Free PSA
☐ Bilirubin	☐ Vaginal	☐ Insured Meets OHIP eligibility criteria
☐ Albumin	☐ Vaginal/Rectal – Group B Strep	☐ Uninsured - Screening Patient responsible for paying
☐ Lipid Assessment	☐ Chlamydia (specify source)	
Includes Cholesterol, HDL-C, Triglycerides, calculated LDL-C & Chol/HDL-C ratio; individual lipid tests may be ordered in the "Other Tests" sections of this form.	Source	**Vitamin D (25-Hydroxy)**
	☐ GC (specify source)	☐ Insured Meets OHIP eligibility criteria: osteopenia; osteoporosis; rickets; renal disease; malabsorption syndromes; medications affecting vitamin D metabolism
	Source	
	☐ Sputum	
☐ Vitamin B12	☐ Throat	
☐ Ferritin	☐ Wound (specify source)	☐ Uninsured - Screening Patient responsible for paying
☐ Albumin/Creatinine Ratio, Urine	Source	
☐ Urinalysis (Chemical)	☐ Urine	**Other Tests**
☐ Ferritin	☐ Stool Culture	
☐ Neonatal Bilirubin:	☐ Stool Ova & Parasites	
Child's age: days hours	☐ Other Swabs/Pus (specify source)	
Clinician/practitioner's phone #:	Source	
	Specimen Collection	
Patient's 24-hour phone #:	Time / Date	
	Fecal Occult Blood Test (FOBT) (check one)	
Therapeutic Drug Monitoring	FOBT (non CCC)	
Name of Drug 1	Colon Cancer Check (FOBT) CCC	
Name of Drug 2	***Laboratory Use Only***	
Time Collected Drug1 (hr)		
Time of Last Dose 1 (hr)		
Time of Next Dose 1 (hr)		
I hereby certify the tests ordered are not for a registered patient of Hope General on an inpatient or outpatient basis		
Signature		

APPENDIX 7.19

Height and Weight Conversion Table

Height			Weight		
Convert Centimetres to Feet and Inches (centimetres × 0.3937 = inches)			**Convert Kilograms to Pounds** (kilograms × 2.2 = pounds)		
CENTIMETRES		**FEET AND INCHES**	**KILOGRAMS**		**POUNDS**
142.00	=	4'8"	0.45	=	1
144.50	=	4'9"	0.91	=	2
147.00	=	4'10"	1.36	=	3
150.00	=	4'11"	1.81	=	4
152.50	=	5'	2.27	=	5
155.00	=	5'1"	2.72	=	6
157.50	=	5'2"	3.18	=	7
160.00	=	5'3"	3.63	=	8
162.50	=	5'4"	4.08	=	9
165.00	=	5'5"	4.53	=	10
167.50	=	5'6"	11.34	=	25
170.00	=	5'7"	22.68	=	50
172.50	=	5'8"	34.02	=	75
175.00	=	5'9"	45.36	=	100
177.50	=	5'10"	49.90	=	110
180.00	=	5'11"	54.43	=	120
183.00	=	6'	58.97	=	130
185.50	=	6'1"	63.50	=	140
188.00	=	6'2"	68.04	=	150
190.50	=	6'3"	72.57	=	160
193.04	=	6'4"	77.11	=	170
195.58	=	6'5"	81.65	=	180
198.12	=	6'6"	86.18	=	190
200.66	=	6'7"	90.72	=	200
203.20	=	6'8"	95.25	=	210

Medical Office Pharmacology

8

LEARNING OUTCOMES

After completing this chapter, you should be able to:

- identify and understand the statutes, regulations, and agencies that control and regulate drugs in Canada
- define key terms in pharmacology
- explain the role of the medical office administrator as it relates to pharmacology
- identify four sources of drugs
- distinguish between a drug's chemical name, its generic name, and its brand/trade name
- identify common drug reference guides and explain how they may be used
- describe two ways drugs may be dispensed, and outline the categories of OTC drugs
- explain the factors that affect the efficacy of a drug
- outline four ways of classifying drugs
- differentiate between the types of drug forms, and identify different types of preparations in solid, semi-solid, and liquid form
- "read" a prescription and understand common abbreviations related to prescriptions
- explain best practices for storing and disposing of drugs

*It is much more important to know what sort of a patient
has a disease than what sort of a disease a patient has.*

—William Osler

Introduction

As a medical office administrator, you will never prescribe or administer medications, yet you will require a working knowledge of pharmacology. You will maintain medications in patients' charts, transcribe medications in reports, be asked questions about medications by patients, and deal with pharmacists and pharmacies. You will also maintain accurate records of medications ordered, dispensed, and disposed of, and be involved in phoning in prescriptions and securing prescription pads for your employer.

To prepare you for these responsibilities, this chapter will provide an overview of legislation governing drugs in Canada, basic drug terminology, the sources and classifications of drugs, abbreviations commonly used in prescriptions, and the basic principles of drug storage and disposal.

Regulation and Control of Drugs in Canada

In Canada, the federal and provincial governments are jointly responsible for the regulation and control of drugs and controlled substances designed for human consumption. Federal legislation covers all drugs and controlled substances, legal and illegal, while provincial legislation governs the dispensing and control of medications.

In this section, we will look at the *Food and Drugs Act*, the *Controlled Drugs and Substances Act*, and the National Drug Schedule.

The Food and Drugs Act

The *Food and Drugs Act* (FDA) is a federal statute that regulates the manufacture, export, import, trade, distribution, advertising, and sale of a range of products, including food, drugs, cosmetics, natural health products, contraceptive devices, health-related devices, and hygiene products.

Among other things, the FDA aims to ensure that products that can affect human health are clearly identified as such, and that the general public does not mistake them for ordinary food or cosmetics. The Act also makes it an offence to make unsubstantiated claims about the efficacy of certain products, such as those used to treat serious diseases and health conditions.

The FDA categorizes information in six schedules, two of which are blank at the time of writing (in the context of legislation, a "schedule" is an appendix containing a list, chart, or other collection of data). The schedules are as follows:

- *Schedule A* lists diseases and conditions to which advertising restrictions apply.
- *Schedule B* lists eight standards approved as sources of information for identifying and classifying drugs.
- *Schedule C* lists radiopharmaceuticals and substances used in their production, the sale of which is restricted.
- *Schedule D* lists substances derived from humans, animals, and micro-organisms that can pose health risks through contamination or other causes (for example, human blood products).

The *Food and Drug Regulations* made under the FDA apply to a wide range of goods, including drugs. Among other things, the provisions set out rules for labelling and packaging, possessing, advertising, and selling various products and substances. The federal Health Products and Food Protection Branch of Health Canada is responsible for drug quality, safety, and efficacy. It regulates the manufacture and importation of drugs for sale in Canada, as well as their distribution, including conditions of sale.

> **DID YOU KNOW?**
>
> The first legislation to register medicines in Canada, and the first step in public protection against drugs administered without medical supervision, was the *Proprietary or Patent Medicine Act*, passed in 1909.

Controlled Drugs and Substances Act

The *Controlled Drugs and Substances Act* (CDSA) is Canada's federal statute for controlling and regulating drug use in Canada. The CDSA classifies drugs into four schedules and establishes offences related to drugs and controlled substances. These include possession, trafficking, importing, exporting, and production. The four main schedules set out by the CDSA are as follows:

- *Schedule I* includes many of the most dangerous drugs, including heroin and cocaine. Because these present the greatest health and social problems, penalties related to these drugs are the most serious.
- *Schedule II* includes marijuana and other forms of cannabis.
- *Schedule III* includes, among other drugs, amphetamines and lysergic acid diethylamide (LSD).
- *Schedule IV* includes, among other drugs, tranquilizers and anabolic steroids. Possessing these drugs is legal with a prescription, but importing, exporting, and trafficking are illegal.

Schedule V of the CDSA covers propylhexedrine (a stimulant related to methamphetamine) and its salts; schedule VI covers substances that are used in the manufacture of other controlled substances; and schedules VII and VIII cover cannabis in certain quantities and forms.

> **DID YOU KNOW?**
>
> Drug trafficking is defined by the United Nations as "a global illicit trade involving the cultivation, manufacture, distribution, and sale of substances, which are subject to drug prohibition laws."

The National Drug Schedule

In an effort to harmonize the control of drugs in Canada, the National Association of Pharmacy Regulatory Authorities (NAPRA) partnered with a Health Canada agency to create a "schedule" for the consistent categorization of drugs. This is known as the National Drug Schedule.

Unlike the CDSA model, which classifies drugs according to their chemical similarity and how they are derived, the National Drug Schedule classifies drugs based on the risk they pose to users:

- *Schedule I drugs* require a prescription and are provided to the public by a pharmacist. Examples: amoxicillin, cannabis, lithium, methadone.
- *Schedule II drugs* are less strictly regulated. They do not require a prescription, but they do require intervention from the pharmacist at the point of sale. These drugs are kept behind the pharmacy counter and have no public access. Examples: codeine in certain preparations, EpiPens.
- *Schedule III drugs* are available without a prescription, but must be sold under the direct supervision of the pharmacist in the self-selection area of the pharmacy. Examples: benzocaine for teething, nystatin for topical use.
- *Unscheduled drugs* can be sold without supervision. The labelling is considered sufficient to ensure the appropriate use of the drug. These drugs are not included in schedules I, II, or III, and may be sold at any retail outlet. Examples: acetylsalicylic acid (ASA), bacitracin for topical use, nicotine patches.

Drug Terminology

As an MA, you will routinely discuss medications with patients, as well as with other health care professionals. For example, the physician may ask you to call a patient and request that she adjust her Coumadin dosage from 0.25 mg every day to 0.25 mg *every other day*, further to lab results of INR levels.

Patients may ask you questions directly. For example, physicians often advise parents to double the first dose of Tempra for infants running a high fever, and a parent may ask you for clarification. In this case, you would advise the parent to determine the initial dose from the medication instructions and then double it for the first dose only, and after that to follow the instructions provided by the physician or those listed on the package.

> **DID YOU KNOW?**
>
> It is believed that the "Rx" on a prescription has its origins in the abbreviation of the Latin word *recipe*, meaning "take"—as in the instruction to take the medication. "Sig" comes from the Latin word *signa*, which means "write." It is medical shorthand to the pharmacist meaning, "Please write these instructions on the label for taking this medication."

An understanding of basic pharmacology terms is essential to your ability to function efficiently and professionally in your interactions concerning patient medications. Table 8.1 lists some common terms you should know.

PRACTICE TIP

MAs may NOT give out medical advice, and this includes advice with respect to dosages and types of drugs. If a patient calls with a question about instructions for taking a drug (the "Rx" or "sig" section of the prescription, explained later in this chapter), you may clarify the instructions. However, if the patient is questioning the dose or has missed a dose and is not sure what to do, either ask the physician and then report back to the patient, or suggest the patient speak directly to a pharmacist. If in doubt, *always* check with the physician.

TABLE 8.1　Common Pharmacology Terms

Term	Definition
Addiction	Addiction denotes the condition when a person becomes physically and/or mentally dependent on the abused drug and needs the drug to function normally. A physical dependence is not necessarily an addiction (e.g., blood pressure medications that cause a physical dependence). The four major groups of substances that frequently cause addiction are (i) narcotics, (ii) sedatives and tranquilizers, (iii) amphetamines, and (iv) alcohol.
	An addiction is usually accompanied by a craving for the drug, loss of control over the amount or frequency of use, a compulsion to use the drug, and continued use despite negative consequences. Frequent, ongoing use of substances can cause changes to the body and brain that may be permanent. (Source: Centre for Addiction and Mental Health)

Term	Definition
Adverse effects	These occur when a side effect becomes severe, and are potentially harmful. Types of adverse effects include: headache, upset stomach, dizziness, dry mouth, nausea, and diarrhea. **1. Overdose:** An overdose may occur if a drug dose is too high, if the person is unusually sensitive to the drug, or if another drug slows the metabolism of the first drug and thus increases its level in the blood. The adverse effects of an overdose are anticipated, since they are simply an extension of the drug's normal therapeutic effects. For example, an overdose of a barbiturate will produce over-sedation because barbiturates produce a sedative effect when taken therapeutically. 　　When an overdose occurs, the logical step is to reduce the dose of the drug. **2. Effects unrelated to the main drug action:** Effects unrelated to the main action of a drug—also called secondary effects—may occur because no drug produces one single effect. Secondary effects may be either beneficial or harmful. For example, the digitalis group of drugs is used to strengthen the heart muscle in patients with congestive heart failure (CHF); however, in many cases these drugs produce nausea, vomiting, and abnormal colour vision, effects that are unrelated to their main action of strengthening the heart. If the secondary effects of a drug are harmful and outweigh the benefit of the drug, the drug will be discontinued. **3. Idiosyncrasy:** A variety of unforeseen adverse effects may result from an individual's particular genetic makeup. For example, a drug may act for excessively long periods of time in a person with a slow metabolism. If the efficacy of the drug is altered due to an idiosyncrasy, the physician will adjust the dosage or change the medication. **4. Allergy:** In persons who are allergic to a particular drug, the first time the drug is administered, it combines with a protein to form a complex known as an antigen. The antigen provokes the body to make an antibody, and the antigen–antibody combination provokes an adverse reaction in the patient—a hypersensitivity to the drug. 　　Allergic reactions can range from mild (e.g., a rash, itching, swelling, wheezing, and/or sneezing) to severe (e.g., anaphylactic shock). A drug that produces an allergic reaction will be discontinued and a different drug substituted.
Average dose	The amount of medication taken to produce effective results with a minimal toxic effect
Dose	The amount of medication to be administered
Drug abuse	Drug abuse refers to the harmful, non-medical use of an illegal drug or the misuse of prescription or over-the-counter drugs with negative consequences. These may include: mood swings; health, behaviour, attitude or personality changes; poor muscle coordination; slurred speech; unusual sleepiness or restlessness; and unexplained absences from work, home, or school.
Habituation	Drug habituation (habit) is a psychological condition resulting from repeated use of a drug. A person may experience a desire to continue taking a drug for the feeling of improved well-being it produces, without the need to increase the dose.
Initial dose	The first dose administered
Lethal dose	The amount of a drug that could or does cause death
Maintenance dose	The dose that keeps the concentration of a drug at a therapeutic level
Maximal dose	The largest amount of a drug that will produce a desired effect without symptoms of toxicity
Side effects	The mildest undesirable effects of a drug that occur in addition to the desired therapeutic effect. Side effects are usually mild and short-lived, and may vary depending on the person's disease state, age, weight, gender, ethnicity, and general health. 　　Common side effects include: nausea, vomiting, dizziness, wheezing, shortness of breath, itching, hives, eye redness, and diarrhea.
Therapeutic dose	The smallest amount that will produce a desired effect
Therapeutic index	The range between the minimal and maximal dosages
Tolerance	Decreased physiological response to a drug in a patient due to continued use. To obtain the desired effect, the dosage of the drug may need to be increased because the patient's body has become used to the drug. 　　Tolerance is usually a feature of addiction.
Toxic effects	Toxic effects result when the level of a drug in the patient's system rises above the therapeutic level to a level of toxicity. If the patient suffers from toxic effects, the drug is actually poisoning the patient. A drug that will negate the effect may be administered. For example, if the drug causing the toxicity is an arrhythmic, an anti-arrhythmic may be given.

Drug Sources

People have always sought cures for illnesses and ways to alleviate pain. In early days, naturally occurring substances were used for their medicinal effect, and today many drugs are still based on natural substances. In addition, a wide range of drugs are produced exclusively using chemical substances, or a combination of natural and chemical substances.

Plants

From earliest times, people have identified the healing properties of various plants. Today, many prescription drugs are still derived from plants. At the recommendation of a pharmacist or physician, self-medication with plants is common. Many people use medicinal plants in combination with synthetic drugs.

In the production of a drug, all or part of the plant (leaves, roots, resin, stems, or fruit) may be used. For example, digitalis drugs, such as digoxin, which are used to stimulate the heart in the treatment of congestive heart failure and atrial fibrillation, are derived from the leaves of a type of the foxglove plant known as *Digitalis purpurea*. The plant is toxic, and in rare cases has been known to cause death. Curare, an extract obtained from a number of tropical American plants, was traditionally used as an arrow poison by South American indigenous people, and today is used in anesthesia to relax skeletal muscles during surgery. The commonly used painkiller, codeine, is derived from the opium poppy.

Animals

Domestic animals also provide fluids, tissues, glands, and organs for drug production. The wool from sheep is used in the production of lanolin, which may be used as a topical treatment for burns and infections, as the base for suppositories, in cosmetics, and even in chewing gum.

Other animal pharmaceuticals include hormone replacement drugs, such as pig hormones, which are used to replace or boost human thyroid production, and cow insulin, which can be taken by people who have diabetes. Premarin, the most popular form of estrogen used in hormone replacement therapy to treat the symptoms of menopause, is derived from the urine of pregnant mares. The blood thinner heparin, widely used in heart surgery and kidney dialysis, is derived from pig intestines.

Minerals

Minerals are inorganic nutrients that occur naturally in rocks and metal ores and form part of a healthy diet. People consume minerals when they eat food grown in mineral-rich soil. Minerals that are essential for humans include sodium, potassium, and magnesium. Although minerals are found in a variety of foods, today's North American diet tends toward foods that are high in calories but low in vitamins and minerals. Many people therefore take supplements of common minerals, such as zinc, iron, and calcium.

Potassium—which is found in unprocessed meats, milk, vine and citrus fruits, and leafy green vegetables—is one mineral that individuals may not ingest from their normal diet and for which they may take a supplement. A low-potassium, high-sodium diet may be one of many factors leading to high blood pressure, hypertension, and cardiovascular disease.

The trace mineral iron is vital to overall good health. The World Health Organization considers iron deficiency the number one nutritional disorder globally, with as many as 80 percent of the world's population suffering from it.

Patients who take certain medications may be in particular need of mineral supplements. For example, stimulant laxatives can reduce calcium absorption, and oral contraceptives may decrease serum magnesium levels.

DID YOU KNOW?

Bismuth minerals, which contain the chemical element bismuth, are used in the common upset-stomach medication Pepto-Bismol.

Synthetic and Semi-Synthetic

Synthetic and semi-synthetic drugs are completely formulated in the laboratory, and can be produced either by combining various chemicals or by combining a mineral, animal, or plant substance with chemicals. In addition, they may be genetically engineered or produced by altering animal cells. Genetically engineered drugs include human and bovine growth hormones and human insulin.

Synthetically produced drugs can be produced in large volumes and are usually less expensive. Examples include diazepam (trade name, Valium), ASA (acetylsalicylic acid; trade name, Aspirin), ibuprofen (Advil), and fluoxetine (Prozac). Synthetic forms of insulin have been available since 1981, and today there is widespread use of insulin produced from genetically modified bacteria and yeast. While malaria drugs were previously produced using plant-based methods that took 15 months, researchers recently engineered a strain of baker's yeast that can produce the drugs on an industrial scale, stabilizing the world's supply and cutting down production time to three months.

Genetic engineering has raised many legal and ethical issues. For example, while stem cell research may one day allow us to grow new arms or legs, and while it is likely that no one would argue this should not be done, what if it were possible to create a complete human being? There is a great deal of potential for abuse in genetic engineering, and the possibility of choosing or creating one's own vision of humanity is not just science fiction.

Drug Names

Most drugs on the market have three names: a chemical name, a generic name, and a brand or trade name. Drugs derived from plants have a botanical name.

Chemical Name

The **chemical name** of a drug denotes its atomic or molecular structure and is given when a new drug is developed or discovered. The chemical name of the anti-anxiety drug lorazepam, for example, is 7-chloro-5-(2-chlorophenyl)-1,3-dihydro-3-hydroxy-2H-1,4-benzodiazepin-2-one.

Because chemical names are so complex, they do not have many practical uses. Researchers usually develop a shorthand to refer to a drug in the early stages. In marketing and clinical uses, drugs are referred to by their generic name, trade name, or both.

Generic Name

The **generic name** of a drug is usually created when the drug is ready for marketing, and remains the same throughout the drug's life. Many generic names are derived from the drug's chemical structure. They also reflect the larger class of drugs to which the specific drug belongs, and suggest the drug's action. For example, drugs in the benzodiazepine class, which are used to treat anxiety and other conditions, usually have the suffix "-pam." The generic name for the trademarked drug Valium is diazepam, while that of Ativan is lorazepam.

It is critical that generic names be unique, to prevent confusion and errors in dispensing and administration. Drug name confusion causes thousands of deaths each year.

Unlike trade names, generic names are not proprietary, meaning, they are not copyrighted and can therefore be used in scientific writing, on labelling, and in educational materials without infringing on copyright. Generic drugs may be manufactured by any number of pharmaceutical companies. They usually cost less than brand name versions of the drug; for example, acetaminophen is cheaper than Tylenol, and ibuprofen is cheaper than Advil, but both perform the same function. A pharmacist may fill a prescription for a medication prescribed by its trade name using a less expensive generic form of the medication unless the doctor specifies no substitution, and many insurance plans cover only the generic form of a drug.

DID YOU KNOW?

In Canada, almost 45 percent of all prescriptions filled by pharmacies use generic drugs, and some hospitals use generic drugs almost exclusively.

Companies may claim that the trade name drug is of better quality than the generic version, and there is some concern that certain generic drugs may not be as effective as their trade counterparts. For example, the Society of Obstetricians and Gynecologists of Canada has recommended that brand name versions of birth control pills be used instead of generic ones, stating that new generic versions may not be as effective. While slight differences often exist (for example, altered absorption and excretion rate and a slightly different therapeutic effect), there is no difference in the actual medicinal component of a generic and trade name drug. Health Canada must approve all drugs sold in Canada, and generic drugs must meet the same strict regulations established by the *Food and Drugs Act* as brand name drugs. In addition, the manufacturer must prove that the active ingredients in the generic drug are as pure, dissolve at the same rate, and are absorbed in the same manner as those in the trade product.

Once a drug has passed a review by Health Canada of its formulation, labelling, and instructions for use, it is issued a drug identification number (DIN). The DIN is a randomly generated, eight-digit number that is unique to a drug product and that permits a manufacturer to market the drug in Canada. DINs are issued for over-the-counter (OTC) drugs as well as prescription drugs. Drug products sold in Canada without a DIN are not in compliance with Canadian law.

Brand/Trade Name

When a pharmaceutical company requests approval for a particular drug, it develops a **brand name** that identifies the drug, such as Viagra, Ativan, or Prilosec. A brand or trade name is the name that the drug is marketed under, and it is owned by the pharmaceutical company; no other company may use it. Brand or trade names are always capitalized, and are registered under the *Food and Drug Regulations*.

For marketing reasons, trade names are usually "catchier" and easier to remember than generic names, and may relate to the intended use or benefits of the drug in a subtle way (names that seem to promise a cure for a particular condition, however, will not be approved). For example, Lopressor (metoprolol tartrate) lowers blood pressure, while Glucotrol (glipizide) controls high blood sugar (glucose levels).

In Canada, brand name drugs have 20 years of patent protection. This means the company that first developed the drug has the exclusive rights to make and sell the drug for 20

PRACTICE TIP

In some patients, side effects or adverse reactions to a generic drug may be due to some of the inactive ingredients used (e.g., fillers, flavours, and dyes), which may differ from those used in the trade form of the drug. If a patient mentions adverse effects to you, suggest that he or she discuss medication options with the physician.

years. During this time, other pharmaceutical companies are prohibited by law from producing the drug. This prohibition is intended to protect the drug manufacturer and aid in reimbursement of the costs of research and development. When the 20-year period is up, other manufacturers can apply to Health Canada to market their own versions of the drug. They must use the same generic name, but may create their own trade name. This is why the same generic drug may be sold under many different trade names. For example, the generic drug fluoxetine is sold as Prozac, Sarafem, and Fontex (among other names).

Table 8.2 lists the brand/trade name(s), generic name, and chemical name for several common drugs.

TABLE 8.2   Brand/Trade Names, Generic Names, and Chemical Names for Selected Drugs

Brand/Trade Names	Generic Name	Chemical Name
Aleve, Anaprox, Naprosyn	naproxen	(S)-6-methoxy-α-methyl-2-naphthaleneacetic acid
Pantoloc, Somac, Protonix	pantoprazole	6-(difluoromethoxy)-2-[(3,4-dimethoxypyridin-2-yl) methylsulfinyl]-1H-benzo[d]imidazole
Tylenol, Tempra	acetaminophen	N-acetyl-p-aminophenol

Botanical Names

Botanical history and medical history have been intertwined from the beginning. The earliest botanists were almost always physicians, and, as noted above, many medicines originated from plant life. Today, drugs are still derived from and named after plants. For example, products derived from the plant *Aloe vera* are used in cosmetics as a moisturizer and to heal sunburn and other skin ailments, and eucalyptus oil from the plant *Eucalyptus globulus* is used in over-the-counter cough and cold medicines and as an analgesic.

Telephone Protocol

The telephone has been the primary method of communication between the patient and the physician's office for over 100 years. Telephone communication provides challenges for both the MA and the patient. An MA is not qualified to give medical or medication advice. While most calls may be handled by the experienced MA, there are calls to which only a nurse or physician may respond.

An MA may reply to calls regarding the following:

- schedule patient appointments, including the reason for the visit
- take personal information to establish a new patient; for example, date of birth, address, current medications, telephone number, insurer (if applicable)
- schedule referrals and patient tests
- provide information on location of referral or tests
- provide information on how to prepare for and what to expect with tests
- edit the chart information—for example, adding an allergy, updating a change in address or telephone number
- confirm medication information—dose, route, frequency of medication, as written in charts

An MA may also take calls from medical laboratories with patient test results and calls from outside professionals.

An MA may *not* reply to the following calls, but will take a message and refer the call to the physician or nurse:

- test results
- a patient requiring medical advice
- a patient returning a call from a physician (unless the physician has left instructions for the MA regarding the call)
- a patient experiencing side effects from medication or other abnormal physical symptoms

SCENARIO 8.1

You receive a phone call from a patient who was given a prescription for the birth control pill Alesse. When she picked up her prescription from the pharmacy, the pharmacist had filled the prescription with a less expensive version of the drug containing the same medicinal ingredients, called Aviane. The pharmacist informed the patient that her insurance covers only the generic drug and not the brand name.

The patient is very upset and calls the office. How can you help her? Does she have a right to the brand name prescription? With whom should she discuss her options?

SCENARIO 8.2

A patient calls the office on a Friday evening to ask for a renewal of her pain medication. You retrieve her chart, check her medication list, and note that the painkiller was prescribed three weeks ago and should have lasted for four weeks. Do you confront the patient about the fact that she is taking more pain medication than prescribed? To whom should this phone call be directed?

SCENARIO 8.3

The pharmacist calls from the local drug store. He is looking at a prescription written by your physician, and he has the following questions:

1. The first drug on the prescription is not recommended for a patient with high blood pressure; would the physician like to amend the prescription?
2. The dosage information on the second drug is illegible. The recommended dose is 25 mg bid—is this the dose requested?

How should the MA handle this phone call? The dose for the second drug is clearly written in the chart. Would it be okay for the MA to confirm the drug dose based on the chart?

Law and Ethics

It is important for a medical professional to understand medical law, ethics, and protected health information as it pertains to current legislation (see Chapter 4). There are two main reasons for medical professionals to study law and ethics: The first is to help you function at the highest professional level by providing competent, compassionate health care to patients, and the second is to help you avoid legal problems that can threaten your ability to earn a living.

In order to understand medical law and ethics, it is helpful to understand the differences between them. A **law** is defined as a rule of conduct or action prescribed or formally recognized as binding or enforced by a controlling authority. Governments enact laws to keep society running smoothly. **Ethics** are defined as moral principles, or the rules that guide our conduct (behaviour), based on our belief of what is right and wrong. For example, in 1969, a bill was passed into law permitting abortion when an application for an abortion was accepted by the majority of a three-person therapeutic abortion committee. However, while the law may approve abortion, many people may be ethically opposed to such procedures.

Standard of Care

As an MA, you are expected to fulfill the standards of the profession for applying legal concepts to practice. According to the American Association of Medical Assistants, MAs should uphold legal concepts in the following ways:

- maintain confidentiality
- practise within the scope of training and capabilities
- prepare and maintain medical records
- document accurately
- use appropriate guidelines when releasing information
- follow employer's established policies dealing with the health care contract
- follow legal guidelines and maintain awareness of health care legislation and regulations
- maintain and dispose of regulated substances in compliance with government guidelines
- follow established risk-management and safety procedures
- recognize professional credentialing criteria
- help develop and maintain personnel, policy, and procedure manuals

Often, laws dictate what medical assistants may or may not do. For example, in some US states, it is illegal for medical assistants to draw blood. No states consider it legal for medical assistants to diagnose a condition, prescribe a treatment, or let a patient believe that a medical assistant is a nurse or any other type of caregiver. In Canada, many physicians' offices do use MAs who have training in phlebotomy to take blood. Phlebotomy requires only a few months of education, so some MAs may wish to take the additional training.

In addition to what is stated by law, you and the physician must establish the procedures that are appropriate for you to perform.

Administrative Duties and the Law

Many of a medical assistant's administrative duties are related to legal requirements. Paperwork for insurance billing, patient consent forms for surgical procedures, and correspondence (e.g., a physician's letter of withdrawal from a case) must be handled correctly to meet legal standards.

Documentation, such as making appropriate and accurate entries in a patient's medical record, is legally important.

PRACTICE TIP

Always have the patient chart with you when helping determine medication because you will need to be aware of every drug the patient is taking to eliminate the other drugs. If the patient is unsure whether he has the right pill, ask whether he receives home care or if there is someone else in the home who might help identify the correct drug. Once you have the information, you will bring it to the attention of the nurse or the physician, who will advise the patient. If neither of these options is available, suggest that the patient go to a pharmacy with the medication, or book an appointment with the physician within 24 hours to review the patient's medications.

Drug Reference Guides

Two common drug reference guides frequently used by MAs in Canada are the *Compendium of Pharmaceuticals and Specialties* (CPS), published by the Canadian Pharmacists Association, and the relevant provincial or territorial drug formulary, such as the *Ontario Drug Benefit Formulary/Comparative Drug Index*.

The CPS can be an invaluable resource. It allows you to search for a drug by its generic or brand name. For example, if you needed to look up diltiazem, you would turn to the Brand and Generic Name Index, where drugs are listed in alphabetical order—if the name appears in light italics, it is a generic name; brand names are written in bold. Once you have found the brand name, you can go to the white pages and look up all the information for that particular medication.

The CPS also contains glossy pages with pictures of all drugs. This is helpful in cases where you must help a patient determine which pill is which. For example, you might call a patient to adjust his Coumadin dosage, but the patient may not know which of the pills in his blister pack is Coumadin.

The CPS contains a Therapeutic Guide, in which drugs are organized by therapeutic use. This may also be useful to MAs. For example, if a patient knows she is on hypertensive medication but does not remember the name and is not sure when it was last prescribed, you can go to the hypertension section and review the drugs listed there or match one to the patient's chart.

There are many other sections to the CPS, such as the Clin-Info for quick reference information and dosing tools, and a list of poison control centres, health organizations, and pharmaceutical manufacturers. The appendices of the book also contain information about Health Canada programs, information about narcotics, and the forms for reporting adverse drug reactions.

A drug formulary serves as a guide for physicians and pharmacists regarding drug products that are eligible for coverage under plans, such as the Ontario Drug Benefit (ODB). A formulary also provides comparative pricing of drug products, and lists drug product interchangeability. The costs of drugs that are eligible under the ODB are covered by the Ministry of Health and Long-Term Care. The ODB program provides coverage for over 3,800 drug products, including nutrition products and diabetic testing agents.

If a drug is not listed in the *Ontario Drug Benefit Formulary/Comparative Drug Index*, it may be covered under the Exceptional Access program on a case-by-case basis by the Ministry of Health and Long-Term Care. The Trillium Drug Program (TDP) provides coverage for prescription drug products listed in the *Ontario Drug Benefits Formulary*, if prescription costs are higher than 4 percent of household income. (See Appendix 8.1: Application for Trillium Drug Program.)

The *Ontario Drug Benefit Formulary* is primarily used by professional health care practitioners, pharmacies, hospitals, and organizations associated with the manufacture, use, and distribution of pharmaceutical preparations. However, MAs should be familiar with what a drug formulary is and the forms required to access these drugs because it is the MA who will assist the patient with completing the forms to obtain the drug benefits and assist the physician with the drugs available.

Dispensing Drugs

There are two methods for dispensing drugs: by a pharmacist, with a prescription; and over the counter by a pharmacist or self-service, without a prescription.

Prescription Drugs

As described above, federal law makes drugs illegal that are dangerous, powerful, or habit forming, except if prescribed by a licensed physician or other qualified health care provider who is to monitor the patient's condition.

A **prescription** is a written or oral order by a licensed physician or other authorized health care professional (e.g., a dentist, midwife, or nurse practitioner) to a pharmacist to supply a certain patient with a particular drug of specific quantity, prepared according to the prescriber's directions. Technically, the pharmacist should dispense drugs only with a written and physically signed script in hand; however, most pharmacies will accept a faxed (but never a phoned-in) prescription for a controlled substance, such as the narcotic morphine.

Over-the-Counter Medications

Over-the-counter (OTC) medications are considered safe for individuals to take without the specific advice of a physician. OTC drugs are available in pharmacies and a variety of retail outlets. Although these drugs do not require a prescription, they may be harmful if used incorrectly, so most provinces have categorized them to provide some control over access.

Drugs that may be obtained without a prescription fall into the following categories:

- *Pharmacy Only: Restricted Areas* (NAPRA Schedule II drugs). Drugs in this category are available only from a pharmacist and are kept behind the counter. Examples: Gravol, syringes, and test strips.

- *Pharmacy Only: Under Supervision* (NAPRA Schedule III drugs). These drugs are available only in pharmacies and are sold in the self-serve section. Medications in this category include those that could present risks to certain people if used without adequate knowledge. Often, these medications have been recommended by a physician. Examples: Tucks for hemorrhoids, and smoking cessation medications.

- *Sold Anywhere* (Unscheduled NAPRA drugs). These medications may be sold in any retail outlet without any professional supervision. Examples: Aspirin, Advil, Preparation H, Monistat.

Most OTC preparations have instructions and recommendations for use clearly outlined on the package label, but additional patient education better ensures correct and safe usage. Non-prescription medications can negatively interact with prescription medications. In addition, there is always the danger that a person who should see a doctor will self-treat with OTC medications (for example, for chest pain, indigestion, or a yeast infection). Patients must be encouraged to have any persistent problems checked out medically.

Drug Efficacy

In prescribing medications, physicians consider the effectiveness of a particular drug. **Efficacy** is the term that describes a drug's effectiveness—does it produce the desired therapeutic effect? In other words, does it work? The term "potency" is often confused with "efficacy." **Potency** describes a drug's strength, which is often measured in milligrams, for example. A potent drug is able to achieve the desired effect in smaller doses. When comparing two drugs that achieve equal results, the drug with the lower dose has a higher potency. They are equally effective.

Drugs are not necessarily always chosen for their effectiveness. There are other factors a physician considers before prescribing a drug for an individual, such as its potential toxicity, side effects, drug interactions, and the duration of the effects.

Person 1
Signature

X

Date (yyyy/mm/dd)

Person 2
Signature

X

Date (yyyy/mm/dd)

Signature 2 – Consent for Canada Revenue Agency (CRA) to release my Income Information to the Ministry

I authorize for the Canada Revenue Agency (CRA) to release to the Ministry of Health and Long-Term Care information from my income tax returns and other required taxpayer information whether supplied by me or a third party. The information will be relevant to, and used solely for the purpose of determining and verifying eligibility, including determining appropriate deductible amounts, and for the administration of the Trillium Drug Program of the Ontario Drug Benefit Program under the *Ontario Drug Benefit Act*, and will not be disclosed to any other person or organization without my approval, except as required or permitted by law. This authorization is valid for the most recently available of the two taxation years prior to signing this consent and each subsequent consecutive taxation year for which assistance under the *Ontario Drug Benefit Act* may be requested and determined. I understand that, if I wish to withdraw this consent, I may do so at any time by writing to the Trillium Drug Program, PO Box 337, Station D, Etobicoke ON M9A 4X3.

Person 1
Signature

X

Date (yyyy/mm/dd)

☐ I decline to give CRA consent and have attached my proof of income, and acknowledge I will need to provide my proof of income each year to renew with TDP.

Person 2
Signature

X

Date (yyyy/mm/dd)

☐ I decline to give CRA consent and have attached my proof of income, and acknowledge I will need to provide my proof of income each year to renew with TDP.

*If the signature is not that of the person listed, include the signatory's name and identity category in the space below, and attach supporting documents, as appropriate.

Categories for Signatory Identification

1. Person's Guardian of property
2. Person's Guardian of the person
3. Person's Attorney under continuing power of attorney for property
4. Person's Attorney under power of attorney for personal care
5. Substitute Decision Maker

Signatory for Person	☐ Person 1	☐ Person 2	☐ Person 3	☐ Person 4

Last Name of Signatory	First Name of Signatory	Identity Category of Signatory (see categories in box above)
		☐ 1 ☐ 2 ☐ 3 ☐ 4 ☐ 5

The Ministry of Health and Long-Term Care collects information about prescriptions to:

- help pharmacists fill their customers' prescriptions safely and effectively,
- review trends, and
- ensure that health programs meet the needs of people in Ontario.

This information is collected under the authority of the *Personal Health Information Protection Act*, 2004, S.O. 2004, c.3, Sched. A (PHIPA) and Section 13 of the *Ontario Drug Benefit Act*, R.S.O. 1990, c.O.10. This information will be used and disclosed to administer the Trillium Drug Benefit Program and the Ontario Drug Benefit Program. It may be used and disclosed in accordance with PHIPA, as set out in the Ministry of Health and Long-Term Care "Statement of Information Practices" which may be accessed at
http://www.health.gov.on.ca/en/common/legislation/priv_legislation/docs/stat_info_practices.pdf.
For more information regarding the collection and use of personal information, write to the Director, Exceptional Access Program Branch, Ministry of Health and Long-Term Care, at 5700 Yonge Street, 3rd Floor, Toronto, ON M2K 4K5 or call 1 800 575-5386.
In Toronto, call 416 642-3038.

3693-87E (2013/12)

APPENDIX 8.2

Classification of Drugs by Action/Function

Drug Class	Action/Function	Examples
Analgesic	Relieves pain.	• controlled or narcotic drugs, such as morphine sulphate (MS Contin) • non-narcotic drugs, such as acetaminophen (Tylenol, Anacin, Atasol, Tempra)
Antacid	Reduces acid in the stomach and GI tract. May be used for dyspepsia (indigestion) or heartburn.	• aluminum hydroxide (Amphojel, Nephrox, Alka-Seltzer) • magnesium carbonate (Maalox, Diavol)
Anxiolytic, anti-anxiety	Reduces feelings of anxiety.	• diazepam (Valium), alprazolam (Xanax), lorazepam (Ativan)
Antiarrhythmic	Controls abnormal heartbeats (arrhythmias) that affect the electrical conduction of the heart.	• amiodarone (Atli-Amiodarone) • verapamil (Isoptin) • propafenone (Rythmol)
Antiarthritic	Interrupts the inflammatory process.	• NSAIDS (non-steroidal anti-inflammatory drugs): Aspirin, Aleve • Celebrex
Antibiotic	Fights bacterial infections. Drugs that arrest bacterial growth in the human body are described as "bactericidal."	• ciprofloxacin (Ciprol) • erythromycin (Erythrocin)
Anticholinergic	Reduces muscle tremor through central action. Improves impaired memory and learning. (Other drugs, such as antihistamines and antidepressants, have anticholinergic properties.)	• benzatropine mesylate (Cogentin)
Anticoagulant	Commonly called blood thinners; given to prevent blood clots. These drugs are often given intravenously following surgery, particularly to patients with a high risk of developing blood clots. These drugs should not be taken with ASA and certain herbal medications, except under the direction of a physician.	• Oral anticoagulant: warfarin (Coumadin) • Parenteral anticoagulant: heparin
Anticonvulsant	Given to prevent, control, or relieve seizure activity, such as in an individual who has epilepsy.	• carbamazepine (Tegretol) • phenytoin (Dilantin
Antidepressant	Used in the treatment and control of depression. Sometimes used to treat chronic pain. Must NOT be taken with St. John's wort, an herbal antidepressant.	• bupropion (Wellbutrin), amitriptyline (Elavil), fluoxetine (Prozac)
Antidiabetic	Used to control diabetes. Antidiabetic medications have different mechanisms. Hypoglycemics are used to stimulate the pancreas to produce insulin. Other medications work to improve the body's use of insulin and decrease the amount of glucose released by the liver.	• Insulin is a parenteral hypoglycemic used for Type 1 or insulin-dependent diabetes • Oral antihyperglycemics, used for the initial stages of Type 2 or non-insulin-dependent diabetes, increase insulin secretion. These include glyburide (Diabeta), repaglinide (Gluconorm), pioglitazone (Actos), and rosiglitazone (Avandia)
Antidiarrheal	Given to stop or control diarrhea.	• loperamide (Imodium)

Drug Class	Action/Function	Examples
Antiemetic	Given to control or prevent nausea and vomiting.	• dimenhydrinate (Gravol); also taken to prevent motion sickness
Antifungal	Used to treat fungal infections, either locally (athlete's foot) or systemically.	• Topical: miconazole nitrate (Monistat), clotrimazole (Canesten), terbinafine (Lamisil) • Oral: ketoconazole (Nizoral)
Antihistamine	Used to relieve allergies. These drugs block histamine, which is released when a person has an allergic reaction. A common side effect is drowsiness.	• diphenhydramine hydrochloride (Benadryl) • loratidine (Claritin)
Antihypertensive	Lowers and/or controls blood pressure. There is a wide variety of antihypertensives on the market, with different modes of action. Some of these medications impede vasocon-striction or cause vasodilation, increasing the ease of blood flow in the body. Others slow the heart rate and decrease the force of the heart's contraction. Others act on a hormone produced by the kidney called angiotensin that affects blood pressure.	• propanolol (Inderal) • lisinopril (Prinivil) • amlodipine (Norvasc) • ramipril (Altace)
Anti-inflammatory	Controls various inflammatory processes in the body, such as joint inflammation. Carries a high potential for adverse effects, especially with long-term use, such as stomach ulcers.	• NSAIDs: ibuprofen (Advil), naproxen (Anaprox)
Antilipemic	Lowers high levels of fatty substances in the blood. Lowers cholesterol.	• atorvastatin (Lipitor) • simvastatin (Zocor) • pravastatin (Pravachol)
Antipyretic	Reduces fever.	• ASA (Aspirin) • acetaminophen (Tylenol)
Antitussive	Controls or relieves coughing. Many of these medications are Schedule I or II medications.	• Novahistine DM Expectorant • Benylin • Dextromethorphan ("DM"), a long-acting disso-ciative anesthetic and depressant that affects serotonin levels and causes hallucinations by separating perception from sensation
Antiviral	Treats viral infections.	• acyclovir (Zovirax) • amantadine (Symmetrel) • oseltamivir (Tamiflu)
Bronchodilator	Used primarily to treat bronchitis and asthma, these medications cause bronchial passages to relax and ease breathing.	• salbutamol (Ventolin)
Cathartic	Broad term for laxatives.	• magnesium hydroxide (Magnalox, Milk of Magnesia) • bisacodyl (Dulcolax)
Contraceptive	Used for birth control. Various vaginal creams and suppositories also fall into this category. May be given as injections or patches.	• Most common oral contraceptives ("the pill") include Triphasil, Min-Orval

Drug Class	Action/Function	Examples
Decongestant	Alleviates sinus and nasal congestion. These medications act by reducing swelling of the nasal passages. 　　Nasal spray and eye drops should be used for only 3 to 7 days. Longer use can trigger a rebound reaction in which stuffiness and swelling increase as the blood vessels enlarge even more than they did before taking the medication. 　　Oral decongestants do not cause the rebound reaction.	• xylometazoline (Otrivin) • pseudoephedrine (Sudafed)
Diuretic	Aids in the excretion of excessive body fluid, which can relieve symptoms of hypertension and congestive heart failure.	• furosemide (Lasix)
Emetic	Used to induce vomiting, such as in the case of overdose.	• ipecac syrup
Expectorant	Liquefies mucus in the bronchi and aids in the expectoration of sputum, mucus, and phlegm. Relieves and suppresses cough.	• guaifenesin (Duratuss G, Mucinex) • potassium iodide (Pima)
Hormone	Used primarily to replace hormones that the body can no longer produce. Hormones are also used to treat symptoms of menopause and in individuals who are seeking a sex change.	• insulin (Humulin) • levothyroxine (Eltroxin, Synthroid)
Hypnotic	Immunosuppressant; suppresses the body's immune system. These drugs are used in the control and treatment of certain autoimmune diseases, rheumatoid arthritis, and systemic lupus erythematosus, in which the body attacks its own organs and tissues. 　　Used to deal with transplant rejection.	• prednisone (Apo-prednisone) • azathioprine (Imuran)
Myotic	Used by ophthalmologists and optometrists to constrict/contract the pupil of the eye. Also used to treat glaucoma.	• pilocarpine (Salagen)
Mydriatic	Dilates the muscles of the eye (pupil), such as for an eye examination. Some are long-lasting (24 h). The client will be very photosensitive and should not drive.	• atropine (Atropen)
Narcotic	Acts on the central nervous system, causing pain relief, stupor, and sleep. In larger doses it will depress the respiratory system. These drugs have a high potential for addiction and abuse and are usually controlled.	• meperidine (Demerol) • oxycodone (OxyContin) • oxycodone + acetaminophen (Percocet)
Purgative	More powerful than routine laxatives; often taken by clients preparing for diagnostic tests, such as colonoscopy.	• sodium phosphate (Fleet Enema, Phospho-Soda)
Steroid	Reduces inflammation and affects the immune system. 　　May be used in treatment for arthritis, asthma, eczema. 　　Can produce severe side effects, including cataracts and weakened bones. Because of this, they are usually taken for the shortest possible period of time.	• Steroidal anti-inflammatory: prednisone (Apo-prednisone)
Vasodilator	Causes blood vessels to dilate and relax, lowering blood pressure.	• hydralazine (Apresoline) • isosorbide dinitrate (Isordil)
Vasopressor	Contracts arteries and capillaries, raising blood pressure. May be used for clients in hemorrhagic shock.	• norepinephrine (Levophed)

Medical Billing

9

LEARNING OUTCOMES

After completing this chapter, you should be able to:

- understand the structure of a physician's billing number
- identify diagnostic and fee (service) codes and explain how they apply to billing
- explain the differences among health claims/health care payment (HCP) claims, Workplace Safety and Insurance Board (WSIB or WCB) claims, and reciprocal medical billing (RMB) claims
- understand electronic data transfer (EDT) and how to process a claim using medical software
- understand the billing cycle, billing due dates, and remittance dates
- understand payment errors and rejections
- understand billing for uninsured services, including discretionary billing, block fees, and third-party billing

FIGURE 9.4 Billing Confirmed and the Fee Received for Service

The diagnostic code shown in this figure is described in writing below the code. Most electronic medical record (EMR) software allows a person to search for the diagnostic code either by number or diagnosis.

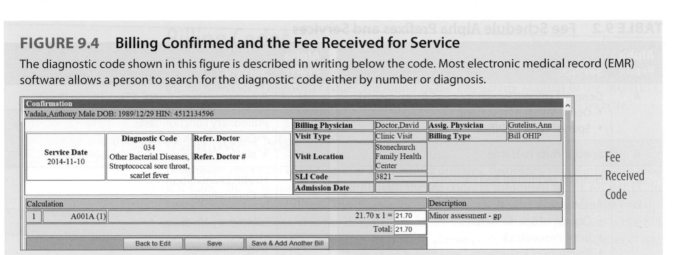

SOURCE: © 2010, Oscar McMaster.

TABLE 9.3 Exceptions to the Diagnostic Code/Fee Code Rule

Family and General Practice	Pediatrics
K017—child	K267—2 to 11 years
K130—adolescent	K269—12 to 17 years
K131—adult age 18 to 64 inclusive	
K132—adult 65 years of age and older	

For a detailed list of exceptions, please refer to Appendix 9.3.

Claims Submission

There are three types of claims a physician submits to OHIP: Health Care Payment (HCP) claim, Workplace Safety and Insurance Board (WISB or WCB) claim, and Reciprocal Medical Billing (RMB) claim. Billing for non-OHIP, third-party claims will be explained later in this chapter.

Health Care Payment (HCP)

A **health claim** or **health care payment (HCP)** is filed for services rendered by a physician or private medical lab to a patient who has Ontario health insurance. When the MA enters the information in an EMR, the payment program would be HCP or OHIP. Some EMRs ask to specify the payee; the payee would be "P" for the physician provider. If the service does not fall under OHIP, the payee would be "S" for the patient.

There are other options available for payments outside of OHIP. For example, in Open Source Clinical Application Resource (OSCAR, a fully featured EMR software program), Interim Federal Health (IFH) is a billing category for federal payments and provides coverage for resettled refugees, refugee claimants, certain persons detained under the *Immigration and Refugee Protection Act*, and other specified groups (see Figure 9.5). Third-party claims will be discussed later in the chapter.

FIGURE 9.5   Billing Type

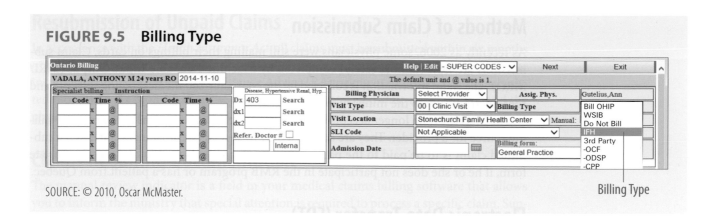

SOURCE: © 2010, Oscar McMaster.

Workplace Safety and Insurance Board (WSIB) Claim

A **Workplace Safety and Insurance Board** (**WSIB** or WCB, for Workers' Compensation Board, an earlier name) claim is for services rendered to patients with Ontario health insurance coverage who have been injured on the job. The payment program choice in this case is WSIB.

If the physician bills any service on a WSIB claim other than a minor or partial assessment, no other assessment can be submitted as an HCP (MOHLTC) claim.

Reciprocal Medical Billing (RMB) Claim

A **reciprocal medical billing (RMB) claim** is used to bill for services rendered by a physician or private medical laboratory to a patient insured under another Canadian provincial health plan outside Ontario, excluding Quebec. The only difference between an RMB claim and an HCP claim is the section on patient information.

The payment program choice in this case is RMB, and the payee is "P" for provider. A physician is not obligated to participate in reciprocal billing and may submit the standard Out-of-Province Claim (Form 0000-80) to receive remuneration (see Appendix 9.4). This form is also used for residents of Quebec and for RMB-excluded services that are OHIP benefits.

Required Patient Information

The necessary patient information for an RMB is as follows:

1. Provincial two-letter code representing the province of the patient's registration
2. Registration number assigned to the patient in his or her province of residence (may be up to 12 characters, without any spaces or special characters)
3. Date of birth in YYYYMMDD format (e.g., 19491225)
4. Patient's surname (up to 13 characters of the patient's last name)
5. Payment program (must be RMB)
6. Payee (must be "P" for provider)
7. Patient's first name (up to six characters)
8. Sex 1 (male) or 2 (female)

PRACTICE TIP

Other than the payment program, the information required to bill a WSIB claim is the same as for HCP claims.

PRACTICE TIP

MAs should always have access to the MOHLTC guides and should take the time to read areas of the guides that apply to billing in their particular office.

Batch Edit Report (EDT Only)

The Batch Edit Report, which is sent within 24 hours of the ministry's receipt of a claims file, acknowledges receipt of each batch submitted, and whether each batch has been accepted or rejected.

Error Reports are normally sent within 48 business hours of claims file submission. Rejected claims can often be resubmitted during the same monthly payment cycle.

Remittance Advice messages are available earlier, usually within the first week of the month, allowing prompt reconciliation of accounts.

Claims Error Report

Claims may be rejected for a variety of error conditions, such as an expired health card or incorrect diagnostic code. Each file submission processed by the ministry will generate an Error Report (if there are errors). Claims rejected on an Error Report are automatically deleted from the payment stream. Rejected claims must be corrected and resubmitted to be processed for payment.

An Error Report provides a list of rejected claims and the appropriate error codes for each claim. Rejected claims may have more than one error code assigned. The MA is responsible for rebilling all items returned with errors. Table 9.4 shows examples of error codes.

TABLE 9.4   Error Report Explanatory Codes

Code	Explanation
02	Incorrect district code—correct and resubmit
03	Date of service does not match OP report—correct and resubmit
04	Special visit premium payable only when submitted with FSC [Financial Status Classification] from the general listings
05	No receipt of supporting documentation requested by MOHLTC

Payment of Claims/Remittance Advice (RA) Report

The physician receives a monthly statement of the approved claims submitted in the previous billing cycle. Both the physician and the MA should carefully review this report to ensure that every claim has been submitted and paid. The **Remittance Advice** (RA) report will include submissions that have been paid in full, underpayments, and rejected claims (see Figure 9.6).

FIGURE 9.6   Sample Remittance Advice (see page 225)

LEGEND:

A Provider Name
B District Office
C Provider Number
D Payment Date
E Page Number
F Provider Account Number
G Patient's Last Name
H Patient's First Name

I Province
J Patient's Health Card Number
K Version Code
L Payment Program
M Claim Number (generated by billing software)
N Service Date
O Number of Services

P Service/Fee Code
Q Fee Submitted
R Amount Paid
S Explanatory Codes
T Page Total
U Total of Previous Pages
V Payment Cheque Number

Continued on next page

FIGURE 9.6   Sample Remittance Advice

A Dr. J.J. Jones   **B** Oshawa (I) B   **C** 0000-123456-01

D

E Page 3

REMITTANCE ADVICE FOR 10 MAY 15

	ACCT'G NO.	PATIENT'S NAME LAST	FIRST	PROV-INCE	REGISTRATION NO.	VER-SION	CONVERTED HEALTH NO.	PAY PGM	CLAIM NO.	SERVICE DATE	NO. OF SERVICES	SERVICE CODE	FEE SUBMIT-TED	AMOUNT PAID	EX CD
01	57079111	Shaw	Olga	On	1234567899	L		HCP	2987654342	150320	01	G310A	6.55	6.55	
02	78956624	Bradford	John	On	9877779933	Q		HCP	B1234577772	150620	01	G303A	8.80	8.80	
03	57085125	Andrews	Geof	On	8933340421	M		HCP	B140823495	150326	01	G700A	4.60	4.60	
04	57009812	Arnold	Anit	On	9725356729			HCP	B1440701277	150408	01	J201A	103.00	103.00	
05	57092264	Kline	Robert	On	8945990023			HCP	B1356788841	150218	01	O310A	6.55	6.55	
06	57081321	Altas	Kait	On	7779356211			HCP	B566892195	150421	01	J201A	103.00	103.00	
07	56912355	Quick	Glen	On	9921456144	Q		HCP	B162889211	150506	01	G313A	8.80	8.80	
08	57092264	Jones	Ralph	On	7753219432	M		HCP	B613215664	150423	01	G310A	6.55	6.55	
09	57699022	Eland	Susan	On	5558210036			HCP	B442172561	150302	01	G313A	103.00	103.00	
10	55532144	Night	Zera	On	3832921443			HCP	B140823178	150318	01	G310A	6.55	6.55	
11	57082166	Archibald	Margaret	On	9727315693			HCP	B1336233997	150222	01	J210A	103.00	103.00	
12	59011125	Anthony	Edward	On	7772457123			HCP	B1992123339	150210	01	G313A	8.80	8.80	
13	57781234	Crisp	Harry	On	4321145679			HCP	B213451677	150108	01	J201A	103.00	103.00	
14	53334891	Brown	Gail	On	7899332145			HCP	B192347892	150307	01	G310A	6.55	6.55	
15	51782311	Lake	Owen	On	9342322431			HCP	B2347891234	150523	01	G313A	103.00	103.00	
												PAGE TOTALS	493.35	493.35	
													4,096.50	4,096.50	

F **G** **H** **I** **J** **K** **L** **M** **N** **O** **P** **Q** **R** **S** **T** **U**

V CHEQUE # 301

INQUIRIES REGARDING OVER-PAYMENTS, UNDER-PAYMENTS, OR NON-PAYMENT MUST BE MADE WITHIN 6 MONTHS OF SERVICE DATE.
FOR LABORATORIES ONLY. FEE SUBMITTED IS TOTAL FEE PAID PER CLAIM

RESOURCES

Billing and Payment Guide for Blended Salary Model (BSM)
Physicians:
http://www.health.gov.on.ca/en/pro/programs/fht/docs/
fht_bsm_physicians_en.pdf

Billing Reference Manual:
http://www.health.gov.on.ca/english/providers/pub/ohip/
edtref_manual/mc_edt_reference_manual.pdf

Diagnostic Codes:
http://www.health.gov.on.ca/english/providers/pub/ohip/
physmanual/download/section_4.pdf

Error Codes Section 4.9 of Physician's Manual:
http://www.health.gov.on.ca/english/providers/pub/ohip/
physmanual/download/section_4.pdf

Explanatory Codes Section 4.11 of Physician's Manual:
http://www.health.gov.on.ca/english/providers/pub/ohip/
physmanual/download/section_4.pdf

Financial Services Commission of Ontario:
http://www.fsco.gov.on.ca/en/forms/Pages/default.aspx

Health Claims for Auto Insurance:
http://hcaiinfo.ca/Health_Care_Facility_Provider/index.asp

Medical Claims Electronic Data Transfer Reference Manual:
http://www.health.gov.on.ca/english/providers/pub/ohip/
edtref_manual/mc_edt_reference_manual.pdf

OHIP Bulletins:
http://www.health.gov.on.ca/en/pro/programs/ohip/
bulletins/4000/bulletin_4000_mn.aspx

Ontario Hospital Association:
http://www.oha.ca

Schedule of Benefits:
http://www.health.gov.on.ca/english/providers/program/
ohip/sob/physserv/physserv_mn.html

Services Requiring Diagnostic Codes:
http://www.health.gov.on.ca/english/providers/pub/ohip/
tech_specific/pdf/5_8.pdf

REVIEW QUESTIONS

True or False?

1. Billing may be submitted only on the 18th of the month.
2. The MA has six months from the date of service to file a billing claim.
3. The first alpha character in a claims error code denotes the type of rejection.
4. When you are looking at the first alpha character in an error code, "V" stands for Assessment Error.
5. EDT stands for *electronic data transfer*.
6. All billing software reports use the same template.
7. Physicians are entitled to charge patients for insured services.
8. A Claims Error Report may contain more than one error code.

Fill in the Blank

1. Private insurance is insurance that is carried outside of _____.
2. The first form to be completed in a WSIB claim is _____.
3. To obtain an Ontario Health Insurance Plan (OHIP) registration number, the physician must have a Certificate of Registration from the College of Physicians and Surgeons of Ontario and a(n) _____.
4. The provider/billing number consists of _____ numbers.
5. To process a billing claim, both the fee code and the _____ must be present (in most cases).

Multiple Choice

1. If a patient is from out of province, the billing type will be

   a. WSIB

   b. HCP

   c. RMB

   d. IFH

2. Which of the following is an uninsured service?

   a. office visit for strep throat

   b. office visit for filling in a work form

   c. office visit for prescription renewal

   d. office visit for referral to a specialist

3. OHIP billing is submitted

   a. once a month

   b. once every two months

   c. as often as the MA would like to submit it

   d. twice a month

4. The last two numbers of the provider/billing number denote

   a physician identification

   b. group/no group status

   c. specialty

   d. locum

5. Which of the selections below describes the four billing error codes?

   a. validity, assessment, eligibility, reciprocal

   b. eligibility, assessment, reciprocal, WSIB

   c. validity, assessment, eligibility, WSIB

   d. eligibility, validity, WSIB, reciprocal

Short Answer

1. Explain and define diagnostic codes versus fee codes.

2. What is a locum?

3. Why should the Remittance Advice be compared with the billing report sent to the MOHLTC?

4. Discuss differences between explanatory codes and error codes.

5. What is a block fee?

HYBRID LEARNING

Midwifery has been regulated in Ontario since 1994. A midwife who orders a pregnancy ultrasound uses the billing codes J159/J459. Using the Schedule of Benefits on the MOHLTC website, explain what these two codes mean and the difference between P1 and P2 codes. What is the remittance amount for each code?

ACTIVITIES

1. Find out the three-digit diagnostic code for each of the following conditions:

Medical Office Procedures: Diagnostic Code Exercise

CONDITION	CODE
Bee sting	
Frigidity	
Neoplasm, unspecified	
Well-baby care	
Vertigo	
Syphilis	
Tapeworm	
Rabies	
Glomerulonephritis	
Gout	
Fanconi syndrome	
Hodgkin's disease	
Abdominal cramps	
Knee joint pain	
Sore throat (not strep)	
Sprained ankle	
Give two examples of visits or procedures that do not require a diagnostic code. Explain what they are.	

2. Complete the following table by filling in the OHIP code and fee from the MOHLTC Schedule of Benefits. The first item is given as an example.

Schedule of Benefits OHIP Code Exercise	OHIP CODE	FEE
Visit		
Adult Annual Health Examination	**A003A**	$ 77.20
Consultation by a Cardiologist		
Family Practice, General Assessment		
Family Practice, Minor Assessment		
Family Practice, Intermediate Assessment		
Repeat Consultation by General Surgeon		
Partial Assessment by Gastroenterologist		
Counselling for 1/2 hour by a Family Physician		
Surgical Procedures/Tests		
Gastroscopy (may include biopsies, photography, and removal of polyps ≤ 1 cm)		
Sigmoidoscopy with Biopsy		
Appendectomy		
Artificial Insemination		
Diagnostic Ultrasound		
Pelvis, Complete (in hospital, physician present)		
Technical Only		
Professional Only		
Total Benefit		
Pregnancy Test		
Pap Test (periodic)		
Immunizations		
MMR (measles, mumps, rubella)		
Influenza		

3. Billing practice using electronic medical record (EMR) software:

   a. In your EMR program, enter the patients from the following chart to the right.

   b. On today's date, enter the following "Reason for Visit" for patients listed. Use the appointment timetable from Chapter 3 if you need a reminder of the typical length of each type of appointment.

   c. Mark the patients "arrived" or "here."

   d. Print the day sheet.

   e. Go to the Billing section of your software and bill each patient.

   f. Using the appointment timetable from Chapter 3, choose the fee/service code for each patient visit. Be sure to include the correct diagnostic codes.

   g. Print out a Billing Summary sheet showing fee code, diagnostic code, and total daily income.

Billing Practice Exercise

Last Name	First Name	Sex	DOB	HC #	Version	Address	City	Prov	Postal Code	Home Phone	Work Phone	Reason for Visit
AHUJA	WINA	F	22/10/1990	4105186870	YX	1013 MACK ST.	KINGSTON	ON	K7K 1B3	613 551-2989	613 556-2058	Diarrhea
JOHNSON	MICHAEL	M	07/03/1937	9503316789	RP	1999 SPADINA CRES.	KINGSTON	ON	K7K 1X1	613 431-9431	613 556-0380	Laryngitis
BENEDETTO	AALIYAH	F	21/10/1945	8551452645	AM	1168 LESLIE DR.	KINGSTON	ON	K7K 1B4	613 551-3231	613 556-1816	Rash on R arm
FATHERS	KOBE	M	11/04/1942	8785546964	GF	17 WOODBINE RD.	KINGSTON	ON	K7K 1V1	613 431-7525	613 556-0979	Swollen L eye
KNIGHT	DIANNA	F	20/05/2012	7853702376		26 GARDINER AVE.	KINGSTON	ON	K7L 1X8	613 431-9863	613 556-0230	Periodic Health Exam
BELL	DANTE	M	16/07/2010	2736376027		9 GOODWIN AVE.	KINGSTON	ON	K7K 1B4	613 551-3224	613 556-1823	Cold
KHURANA	LODI	F	22/10/1990	2560914414	L	121 HILL ST.	KINGSTON	ON	K7L 1X7	613 431-9793	613 556-0265	LN treatment
BELFORD	ANTHONY	M	29/03/1971	9261800057	DY	201 QUEEN ST.	KINGSTON	ON	K7K 1B3	613 551-3216	613 556-1831	Epididymitis
BATTAGLIA	LAURA	F	16/06/1995	1077394714	VP	64 KEEL ST.	KINGSTON	ON	K7K 1A5	613 551-3178	613 556-1869	Strep throat
BAHEN	KOB	M	21/03/2012	8019718025	NG	1988 HWY 2 EAST	KINGSTON	ON	K7K 1B6	613 551-3105	613 556-1942	Earache
LACHAPELLE	KENDRA	F	09/08/2004	7310302828	VE	196 ONTARIO ST.	KINGSTON	ON	K7L 1Y1	613 555-9989	613 556-0178	Stomach cramps
IRVING	TONY	M	03/09/1981	7809619278		37 VICTORIA CRES.	KINGSTON	ON	K7K 1W8	613 431-9311	613 556-0428	Allergy shot
DUNCAN	AUTUMN	F	11/09/2000	4462651052	WF	87 BADER LANE	KINGSTON	ON	K7K 1T7	613 431-7213	613 556-1091	Hair falling out
ELIAS	ETHAN	M	24/06/1960	6599368146		206 PARK ST.	KINGSTON	ON	K7K 1T9	613 431-7354	613 556-1039	Swollen calf
JONES	EMMA	F	25/06/1997	4135443986	WR	8 KENSINGTON AVE.	KINGSTON	ON	K7K 1X1	613 431-9543	613 556-0351	Pap
CZESTIAKOW	STEPHAN	M	14/10/1950	8439893317		12 ENSON ST.	KINGSTON	ON	K7K 1S9	613 431-6601	613 556-1274	Prostate
CAMPBELL	HAILEY	F	28/05/2011	7037337594	GL	105 GROVE RD.	KINGSTON	ON	K7K 1J4	613 551-3501	613 556-1546	Pinkeye
ESMAEILI	MYA	F	03/07/1947	5608648050		17 BROOK ST.	KINGSTON	ON	K7K 1T9	613 431-7472	613 556-1010	Flu
GENEAU	CINDY	F	19/10/1976	4697793927	MN	86 MACLEAN ST.	KINGSTON	ON	K7K 1V8	613 431-8111	613 556-0818	Headaches
DEMAINE	KENDALL	M	21/03/2012	5584451446	TP	21 TORONTO ST.	KINGSTON	ON	K7K 1T3	613 431-6856	613 556-1197	Earache

APPENDIX 9.1

Provincial/Territorial Billing Guides

Province/Territory	Billing Guide	Link
Alberta	Schedule of Medical Benefits (SOMB)	www.health.alberta.ca/professionals/somb.html
British Colombia	Ministry of Health—Medical Services Commission	www.health.gov.bc.ca/msp/infoprac/physbilling/payschedule/index.html
Manitoba	Manitoba Health	www.gov.mb.ca/health/manual/index.html
New Brunswick	New Brunswick Physicians' Manual	www2.gnb.ca/content/gnb/en/departments/health/healthprofessionals.html
Newfoundland and Labrador	Physician's Information Manual	www.health.gov.nl.ca/health/mcp/providers/index.html
Northwest Territories	NWT Health Care Plan	www.hss.gov.nt.ca/health/nwt-health-care-plan
Nova Scotia	Nova Scotia Medical Services Insurance	http://novascotia.ca/dhw/
Nunavut	Same as NWT	
Ontario	Ministry of Health and Long-Term Care	www.health.gov.on.ca/english/providers/program/ohip/sob/sob_mn.html
Prince Edward Island	Master Agreement between the Medical Society of Prince Edward Island and the Government of Prince Edward Island and Health PEI	www.gov.pe.ca/photos/original/doh_masteragree.pdf
Quebec—General Practitioners	Manuel des Médecins Omnipracticiens	www.ramq.gouv.qc.ca/fr/professionnels/medecins-omnipraticiens/manuels/Pages/facturation.aspx
Quebec—Specialists	Same as Quebec—General Practitioners	
Saskatchewan	Saskatchewan Health	www.health.gov.sk.ca/Ministry-overview
Yukon	Payment Schedule for Yukon: Insured Health Services	www.hss.gov.yk.ca/pdf/physicianfeeguide.pdf

APPENDIX 9.2

Provider Specialty Codes

This is a list of specialties or disciplines recognized by the Royal College of Physicians and Surgeons of Canada relevant to services covered under the Ontario Ministry of Health and Long-Term Care.

Specialty Code	Specialty
00	Family Physician
01	Anesthesia
02	Dermatology
03	General Surgery
04	Neurosurgery
06	Orthopedic Surgery
07	Geriatrics
08	Plastic Surgery
09	Cardiovascular and Thoracic Surgery
12	Emergency Surgery
13	Internal Medicine
18	Neurology
19	Psychiatry
20	Obstetrics and Gynecology
22	Genetics
23	Ophthalmology
24	Otolaryngology
26	Pediatrics
28	Pathology
29	Microbiology
30	Clinical Biochemistry
31	Physical Medicine
33	Diagnostic Radiology
34	Therapeutic Radiology
35	Urology
41	Gastroenterology
47	Respiratory Disease
48	Rheumatology
60	Cardiology

APPENDIX 9.3

Services Requiring Diagnostic Codes and Exceptions—Ontario

Fee Schedule Code	Exceptions
A—A	A331A, A335A, A585A, A903A, A990A, A991A, A994A, A995A, A996A, A997A
B—A	B990A–B997A
C—A	C101A, C109A, C110A, C335A, C585A, C903A, C990A, C997A
D—A	
E015A, E100A to E399A, E570 to E687A	
F—A	
G391A to G395A, G400A to G402A, G405A to G407A, G423A, G424A, G521A to G523A, G557A to G559A, G600A to G602A, G610A, G611A, G620A, G621A, G631A, G632A, G634A, G635A, G800A to G805A	
H—A	H001A, H007A, H106A, H110A, H112A, H113A, H261A, H267A

APPENDIX 9.4

Out-of-Province Claim (Form 0000-80)

> ## Ontario
> **Ministry of Health and Long-Term Care**
>
> **Out-of-Province/Country Claim Submission**
>
> - Do not submit receipts for prescription drugs as they are not an insured Ontario Health Insurance Plan (OHIP) benefit.
> - Complete, sign and return this form with your *original* detailed statement that gives a complete breakdown of all charges to a Ministry of Health and Long-Term Care office. Keep copies for your records.
> - If the *original* statement is not in English or French, for accounts:
>   - Under $1000 Canadian, a non-certified translation with a signed statement is acceptable.
>   - $1000 and over, a certified translation is required.
> - If the other criteria for payment set out in the *Health Insurance Act* and Regulations are met, the ministry will pay the amount payable under the Act to an eligible hospital or health facility *directly* upon receipt of an itemized invoice and the signed authorization and direction (see below). The ministry will not make payment directly to an out-of-country physician.
> - If the other criteria for payment set out in the *Health Insurance Act* and Regulations are met, the ministry will pay the amount payable under the Act to the client *directly* for **hospital** or **physician** charges upon receipt of an itemized invoice and *original proof of payment*.
> - Accounts must be submitted within 12 months from date of service. Please allow 6–8 weeks for payment. All payments will be in Canadian funds.
>
> ### Patient Information
>
> | Health Number | Version | Patient's Last Name | First Name |
> |---|---|---|---|
>
> Date of Birth — year month day | Sex ☐ Male ☐ Female | Telephone No. (home) ( ) | Telephone No. (business) ( )
>
> Mailing Address Street Name | City | Province | Postal Code
>
> Residence Address Street Name | City | Province | Postal Code
>
> Date of Departure from Ontario — year month day | Date of Return to Ontario — year month day | Country/Province Where Treatment Provided | Type of currency paid
>
> In the previous 12 month period, have you been absent from Ontario for a period of more than 212 days? ☐ No ☐ Yes ▶ | If yes, provide details.
>
> Are you covered by any travel/supplementary insurance? ☐ No ☐ Yes ▶ | If yes, name of insurance company | Policy Number
>
> ### Treatment Information *(Complete this section in full)*
>
> Was this treatment required due to a condition which arose outside Ontario, was acute and unexpected, and required immediate treatment? ☐ Yes ☐ No
>
> Reason for Visit/Diagnosis *(nature of illness)* | Type of Treatment Received
>
> Place of Treatment ☐ Office ☐ Home ☐ Hospital ☐ Other *(specify)*_____ | Treatment Date — year month day | Time of Treatment : ☐ A.M. ☐ P.M.
>
> ### Hospital Information
>
> Hospital Name | Admission Date — year month day | Discharge Date — year month day
>
> Hospital Address | Please Check (✓) One ☐ inpatient ☐ outpatient
>
> **Knowingly providing false information is an offence punishable by fine and/or imprisonment. The information given on this form is true and accurate.**
>
> Signature of Patient/Guardian | Date
> X
>
> ### Authorization and Direction *(The ministry will pay the amount payable by OHIP directly to an eligible hospital or health facility upon receipt of an itemized invoice and the signed authorization.)*
>
> I, _____ authorize and direct the Ministry of Health and Long-Term Care to pay the
> Name of Patient *(print)*
>
> amount of my hospital / health facility bills that are payable by OHIP directly to _____
> Name of Hospital/Health facility *(print)*
>
> Signature of Patient/Guardian | Date
> X
>
> By submitting this form to the Ministry, you are consenting to the Ministry's use of the information contained in this form for the purpose of assessing, verifying and monitoring eligibility for payment for OHIP insured services and for the proper administration of the *Health Insurance Act* and other Acts/programs administered by the Ministry. For information about collection practices, call 1 800 268–1154, in Toronto (416) 314–5518, or by mail to your local Ministry of Health and Long-Term Care Office.
>
> **For more information, contact a claims processing office (collect calls accepted) or visit our web site at: www.health.gov.on.ca**
>
> **London**
> 130 Dufferin Ave., 4th Fl., N6A 5R2
> 519 873–1303
>
> **Ottawa**
> 75 Albert St., 7th Floor, K1P 5Y9
> 613 237–9100
>
> **Thunder Bay**
> 435 James St. S., Suite 113, P7E 6T1
> 807 475–1353
>
> 0951–84 (2014/02) ©Queen's Printer for Ontario, 2014   ©Imprimeur de la Reine pour l'Ontario, 2014   7530–4568

APPENDIX 9.5

Claims Flagged for Manual Review (Form 2404-84)

Ontario

Ministry of Health
and Long-Term Care

Ministère de la Santé
et des Soins de longue durée

Claims Flagged for Manual Review

Demandes de règlement à traiter manuellement

This form is for manual review only. DO NOT use this for inquiries. Submit the completed form(s) with your disk/tape.
Ce formulaire porte uniquement sur le traitement manuel des demandes. Veuillez NE PAS l'utiliser pour demander des renseignements. Remettez le/les formulaire(s) dûment rempli(s) accompagné(s) de votre disquette/cassette.

A. Provider Information / Renseignements sur le fournisseur ou la fournisseuse

Provider/Group Number / Nº du/de la fournisseur(euse) / du groupe   Provider's Name / Nom du fournisseur ou de la fournisseuse

Office Contact Name / Nom de la personne contact du bureau   Office Contact Phone No. / Nº de tél. de la personne contact
(   )

B. Patient Information / Renseignements sur le patient ou la patiente

Health Number / Numéro de carte Santé   Patient's Name / Nom du/de la patient(e)   Date of Birth / Date de naissance
yyaa   mm   dj

Service Date / Date du service   Service Code / Code du service   Account Number *(if available)* / Nº de compte *(si disponible)*

C. Detention Time *(including report and time spent with patient)*
Temps consacré au cas *(y compris le temps passé à la rédaction d'un rapport et en compagnie du patient ou de la patiente)*
K001A: Time spent exclusively with the patient following the consultation/assessment. Refer to the Schedule of Benefits, General Preamble for conditions and limitations.
K001A : Temps passé exclusivement avec le/la patient(e) a près de la consultation ou l'évaluation. Les conditions et les restrictions sont indiquées dans le préambule général de la liste de prestations.

Assessment Start Time / Heure du début de l'évaluation	Assessment End Time / Heure de la fin de l'évaluation
Hr. / h	Hr. / h
Detention Start Time / Heure du début du temps consacré au cas	Detention End Time / Heure de la fin du temps consacré au cas
Hr. / h	Hr. / h

K101A: Time of Departure Patient(s) / Heure du départ du (des) patient(s)	Time of Arrival / Heure d'arrivée
Hr. / h	Hr. / h
K111A: Boarding Time Patient(s) / Heure d'embarquement du (des) patient(s)	Disembark Time / Heure de débarquement
Hr. / h	Hr. / h
K112A: Return Without Patient(s) / Retour sans patient(s) ou patiente(s) Time of Departure / Heure de départ	Time of Arrival / Heure d'arrivée
Hr. / h	Hr. / h
K102A: Time of Departure / Heure de départ	Time of Arrival / Heure d'arrivée
Hr. / h	Hr. / h
K102A (Return) / (Retour) : Time of Departure / Heure de départ	Time of Arrival / Heure d'arrivée
Hr. / h	Hr. / h

Critical care with report including time spent with patient when providing resuscitation *(indicating actual beginning and ending time)*
Soins d'urgence avec rapport, y compris le temps passé à réanimer le/la patient(e) *(indiquer les heures exactes de début et de fin)*

Start Time / Heure du début	End Time / Heure de la fin
Hr. / h	Hr. / h

D. Independent Consideration *procedures or complex medical procedures, include an operative report and comparision with a listed service in terms of scope, difficulty and value.*
Interventions prises en considération *séparément ou interventions complexes, y compris un rapport sur l'opération et une comparaison avec un service faisant partie de la liste sur le plan de l'étendue, de la difficulté et de la valeur.*

For other fee schedule codes requiring additional documentation, please refer to the Schedule of Benefits, General Preamble.
Pour d'autres codes du fichier des honoraires nécessitant des documents supplémentaires, se reporter au préambule général de la liste de prestations.

E. Multiple visits same day: *(state clinical reason)* / **Visites multiples le même jour :** *(indiquer la raison d'ordre clinique)*

Code	Time of 1st Visit / Heure de la 1re visite	Reason / Raison
	Hr. / h	
Code	Time of 2nd Visit / Heure de la 2e visite	Reason / Raison
	Hr. / h	
Code	Time of 3rd Visit / Heure de la 3e visite	Reason / Raison
	Hr. / h	

F. Other: / Autre :

Instructions on reverse / Instructions au verso ➞

2404–84 (07/09)   ©Queen's Printer for Ontario, 2007   © Imprimeur de la Reine pour l'Ontario, 2007   7530–5248

APPENDIX 9.6

Request for Approval of Payment for Proposed Surgery (Form 0691-84)

> **Ontario**
>
> Ministry of Health
> and Long-Term Care
>
> Ministère de la Santé
> et des Soins de longue durée
>
> **Request for Approval of Payment for Proposed Surgery**
>
> **Demande d'approbation de réglement de frais d'actes chirurgicaux proposées**
>
> **Patient Identification / Identification du malade**
>
> Patient's last name and initials / Nom de famille et initiale(s) du malade
>
> Patient's address / Adresse du malade
>
> Health Number / Numéro de carte Santé   Version code   Sex/Sexe   M   F
>
> Patient's first name / Prénom du malade   Date of birth / Date de naissance   yr./an.   mo.   day/jr.   Postal Code / Code postal
>
> **Surgery Details / Renseignements sur l'intervention chirurgicale**
>
> Name and address of hospital / Nom et adresse de l'hôpital
>
> Date of admission (if known) / Date d'admission (si connue)   Proposed fee / Honoraires envisagés
>
> Diagnosis and proposed procedure / Diagnostic et acte envisagé
>
> Medical indication for surgery / raisons médicales justifiant l'intervention chirurgicale
>
> Reason for referral outside Ontario / Raison de la recommandation d'un spécialiste á l'extérieur de l'Ontario
>
> Surgeon's and/or referring physician's name in full
> Nom et prénoms du médecin qui adresse le malade ou/et du chirurgien
>
> Surgeon's and/or referring physician's address / Adresse du médecin et/ou du chirurgien nommés
>
> Surgeon's and/or referring physician's Ministry of Health and Long-Term Care identification number
> Numéro d'identification Ministère de la Santé et des Soins de longue durée du médecin et/ou du chirurgien nommés
>
> Surgeon's and/or referring physician's signature
> Signature du médecin et/ou du chirurgien nommés   Date   Postal Code / Code postal
>
> **Ministry of Health and Long-Term Care Assessment / Évaluation par le Ministère de la Santé et des Soins de longue durée**
>
> 1 and 2 pertain on condition that Ontario Health coverage is in effect on date of service.
> Les remarques 1 et 2 ne sont à considérer que si la Protection-santé de l'Ontario est en vigueur à la date ou les soins sont dispensés.
>
> ☐ 1. Approved for benefits as submitted
> 1. Règlement approuvée sans modification
>
> ☐ 2. Approved as amended
> 2. Approuvé avec modifications
>
> ☐ 3. Not an eligible benefit
> 3. Intervention non couverte
>
> Comments/Remarques
>
> This authorization is valid for one year after date of approval.
> La présente autorisation est valide pour un an à compter de la date d'autorisation.
>
> Signature for Ministry of Health and Long-Term Care
> Signature au nom du Ministère de la Santé et des Soins de longue durée   Date
>
> **Instructions to surgeons/physicians:**
> 1. Forward all copies of this form to Medical Consultant c/o your Ministry of Health and Long-Term Care office.
> 2. Please advise Assistant and Anaesthetist of status of claim. (that Approval has to be requested).
> 3. Return your copy of this form with your claim card if request is approved.
> 4. Please print or type, you are making 4 copies.
>
> **Instructions au chirurgien/médecin :**
> 1. Envoyez toutes les copies de cette formule au médecin-conseil, aux soins du bureau du Ministère de la Santé et des Soins de longue durée.
> 2. Veuillez aviser l'assistant et l'anesthésiste qu'une demande d'approbation est en cours.
> 3. Si la demande est approuvée, renvoyez votre copie de la formule avec votre carte de demande de règlement.
> 4. Veuillez dactylographier ou écrire en lettres moulées – vous faites quatre copies.
>
> **(See reverse / Au verso)**
> 0691–84 (2000/03)
>
> Part 1 – Surgeon   Part 3 – Ministry of Health and Long-Term Care   Part 4 – Hospital
> Copie 1 – Chirurgien   Copie 3 – Ministère de la Santé et des Soins de longue durée   Copie 4 – Hôpital
> Part 2 – Patient
> Copie 2 – Malade   7530–4239

APPENDIX 9.7

Remittance Advice Inquiry (Form 0918-84)

Ontario

Ministry of Health and Long-Term Care

Ministère de la Santé et des Soins de longue durée

Remittance Advice Inquiry
Demande de renseignements
(Avis de règlement)

Confidential when completed
Renseignements confidentiels

Important

A. State your Provider and Group number.
B. State your name and address.
C. Retain **pink** copy for your records.
D. Send white and yellow copies to your **Ministry of Health and Long-Term Care Office.**

A. Inscrivez votre numéro de fournisseur et votre numéro de groupe.
B. Inscrivez votre nom et adresse.
C. Gardez la copie **rose** pour vos dossiers.
D. Envoyez les copies blanche et jaune à votre **bureau du ministère de la Santé et des Soins de longue durée.**

Instructions

1. Use this form to itemize **under** or **over** payments ONLY.
2. Claims outstanding for two payment cycles (remittances) after submission should be re-submitted if no advice received.
3. Inquiries on claim payments should be made within **one** month of receipt of remittance advice.
4. Submit all inquiries from one remittance advice at the same time.

1. N'utilisez cette formule **QUE** pour dresser la liste des paiements **insuffisants** ou **excédentaires.**
2. Les demandes de règlement toujours en souffrance après deux périodes de paiement doivent être soumises à nouveau si on n'a reçu aucun avis.
3. Les demandes de renseignements sur les paiements doivent être faites moins d'un mois après réception de l'avis de règlement.
4. Soumettre en une seule fois les demandes relatives au même avis de règlement.

Date of Remittance Advice
Date de l'avis de règlement

Provider / Group number
Numéro de fournisseur/groupe

Provider/Group name / Nom du fournisseur groupe

Address /Adresse

Postal Code / Code postal

Telephone number / N° de téléphone

Date of inquiry / Date de la demande

		U.R. / A.É.
Under review – you will be advised	A l'étude – on vous avisera	
Paid correctly according to our records	Payé correctement selon nos dossiers	P.C.
Adjustment required – being processed	Redressement requis –présentement en cours	A.R. / R.R.

U.P. – underpayment   O.P. – overpayment
P.I. – paiement insuffisant   P.E. – paiement excédentaire

Claim information / Renseignements (demande de règlement)	U.P. Q.P. P.E	Provider/group remarks / Observations du fournisseur/groupe	Office use only / Réservé au bureau	Code
Health No. / N° de carte Santé				
Claim No. / N° de la demande de règlement				
Fee schedule code / Code du barème des droits				
Date of service / Date du service Y/A MM D/J				
Fee submitted / Droits présentés				
Surname / Nom de famille First name / Prénom				
Date of birth / Date de naissance Y/A MM D/J				
Accounting No. / N° de compte				
Health No. / N° de carte Santé				
Claim No. / N° de la demande de règlement				
Fee schedule code / Code du barème des droits				
Date of service / Date du service Y/A MM D/J				
Fee submitted / Droits présentés				
Surname / Nom de famille First name / Prénom				
Date of birth / Date de naissance Y/A MM D/J				
Accounting No. / N° de compte				
Health No. / N° de carte Santé				
Claim No. / N° de la demande de règlement				
Fee schedule code / Code du barème des droits				
Date of service / Date du service Y/A MM D/J				
Fee submitted / Droits présentés				
Surname / Nom de famille First name / Prénom				
Date of birth / Date de naissance Y/A MM D/J				
Accounting No. / N° de compte				

Name of clerk (print)
Nom du commis
(Lettres moulées)

Telephone
Téléphone

Date returned to provider/group
Retournée au fournisseur/groupe le

0918–84 (2000/01)   ©Queen's Printer for Ontario, 2000   ©Imprimeur de la Reine pour l'Ontario, 2000   7530–4240

APPENDIX 9.8

Uninsured Medical Services, Including Associated Costs Not Covered by OHIP

Procedures	
Treatment of warts/lesions with liquid nitrogen	$20–$55
Single cosmetic lesion removal (nevus, verruca, keratosis)	$60
Two lesions	$75
Three or more lesions	$110
Vaccines	
Dukoral	$45
Hepatitis A	$60
Hepatitis A Junior	$35
Hepatitis B	$25
Hepatitis B Junior	$20
Menactra/Menveo/Nimenrix	$125
Menomune	$130
Twinrix Adult	$70
Twinrix Pediatric	$35
Vivotif (Oral Typhoid)	$40
Vivaxim (Hep A–Typhoid)	$95
Zostavax	$195
Varivax	$70
Rotarix	$97.50
Bexsero	$145
Gardasil—Current University of Ottawa Student	$150
Gardasil—Non-University of Ottawa Student	$165
Cervarix—Current University of Ottawa Student	$100
Cervarix—Non-University of Ottawa Student	$120
Prevnar	$115
Influenza	$10
FluMist	$25

Injections	
Durolane	$350
Suplasyn	$250
Cortisone	$25
Kenalog (40 mg/mL)	$10
Equipment	
Elastic bandages	$10
Theraband strip	$5
IUD (intra-uterine device)	$175
Pregnancy test	$10
Splint	$10
Needles (acupuncture, ART)	$10
Respicare tube inhalation	$12
Forms	

Please note that your provider may charge a fee in addition to those listed below to complete your forms that is commensurate with the time it takes to complete the form.

Occupational Health Report (Health Canada)	$40
Attending Physician Statement (no exam required)	$125
Medical Certificate—UOHS Standard Form	$20 ($15 for students)
Medical Certificate—Other	Variable rate

Copy and transfer of chart	
Complete digital copy of chart	$45
Digital copy of chart to insurance company	$125
Portion of a chart reviewed by a physician ($39.45 for pages 1–5 and $1.55 per page thereafter)	$39.45
Photocopies	At discretion of physician

Third-Party Physical (exam and report)	
Third Party includes: Employers, Insurance Companies, Athletic Clubs, Institutions, Summer Camps, etc.	$160

Immigration Canada physical (exam and report)	
0 to 10 years	$250
11 to 59 years	$280
60 years and over	$300

Physiotherapy visits	
Physio initial assessment	$90
Physio follow-up	$60

Visit Fee	
General (A3) (does not include fees for report)	$120
Intermediate (A7)	$60
Minor (A1)	$40
Patients without a valid health card	$60
Quebec patients (RAMQ)	$20
Civil Aviation physical (exam and report)	$160

Prescription Renewals or Referrals	
Book an appointment to see your provider to request a prescription renewal or referral	No fees
University of Ottawa and Saint Paul University students, UOHS patients granted financial exemption	No fees
Pharmacy faxes your prescription renewal request to your provider	$20
Request for a referral for massage therapy, physiotherapy, etc. without a visit to your provider	$20

Vasectomy	
Quebec (RAMQ) patient fees not covered by Health Card	$100

Missed Appointments	
Regular	$30
Physical	$60
Dietitian	$45
Psychiatry (Non-Student)	$100
Psychiatry (Student)	$50

Sports medicine consultation	$60
Sports medicine follow-up	$30
Sports medicine—MVA, WSIB, concussion, or back	$120
Civil Aviation physical	$75
Physio initial assessment	$90
Physio follow-up	$60
Travel medicine consultation	$50

Listed below are the travel medicine fees that are not covered by OHIP: Please note that these fees are subject to change without notice. (Last update: April 2014)

Travel Medicine Consultation	
Travel visit—1st patient	$60
Travel visit—each additional patient living at the same address and going to the same destination	$50

Travel Vaccines	
Tuberculosis test for travel (includes injection, follow-up with nurse, result card)	$40
Dukoral	$45
Rabies	$230
Japanese encephalitis	$245
Yellow fever	$150
Hepatitis A	$60
Hepatitis A Junior	$35
Hepatitis B	$25
Hepatitis B Junior	$20
Menactra/Menveo/Nimenrix	$125
Twinrix Adult	$70
Twinrix Pediatric	$35
Vivotif (Oral Typhoid)	$40
Vivaxim (Hep A–Typhoid)	$95
Deltamethrin-impregnated bed nets	$56.44
Water purification drops	$19.95
Water bottle with microbiological filter	$29.95
IAMAT Guide to Healthy Travel	$15
Travel booklet (replacement)	$5

SOURCE: University of Ottawa, www.uottawa.ca/health/fees/.

APPENDIX 9.9

WSIB Health Professional's Report (Form 8)

wsib cspaat ONTARIO

Fax To:
416-344-4684
OR 1-888-313-7373

Claim Number (If known)

8 **Health Professional's Report (Form 8)**

A. Patient and Employer Information - (Patient to complete Section A)

Last Name	First Name	Init.	Sex ☐M ☐F
Address (no., street, apt.)	City/Town	Prov. **ON**	Postal Code
Telephone	Social Insurance No.	Date of Birth dd mm yyyy	Language ☐Eng. ☐Fr. ☐Other
Employer Name			

The Workplace Safety and Insurance Board (WSIB) collects your information to administer and enforce the Workplace Safety and Insurance Act. The Social Insurance Number may be used to identify workers and to issue income tax information statements as authorized by the Income Tax Act. Questions should be directed to the decision maker responsible for your file or toll free at 1-800-387-5540.

B. Incident Dates and Details Section

1. How did the injury/reinjury or illness occur at work?

Occupation

Date of incident/or when did the symptoms start?   dd   mm   yyyy

C. Clinical Information Section - (Please check all that apply)

1. Area of Injury/Illness

☐ Brain	☐ Ears	☐ **Upper back**		Left ☐	Right ☐ **Shoulder**	Left ☐	Right ☐ Wrist	Left ☐	Right ☐ Hip	Left ☐	Right ☐ Ankle
☐ Head	☐ Teeth	☐ **Lower back**		☐ Arm		☐ Hand		☐ Thigh		☐ Foot	
☐ Face	☐ Neck	☐ Abdomen		☐ Elbow		☐ Fingers		☐ Knee		☐ Toes	
☐ Eyes	☐ Chest	☐ Pelvis		☐ Forearm				☐ Lower Leg			
☐ Other:											

2. Description of Injury/Illness Physical Examination Findings

☐ Pain at rest/Night Pain

Pain Rating Scale
0 1 2 3 4 5 6 7 8 9 10

Exposure/Illness

☐ Abrasion	☐ Disc Herniation	☐ Inflammation	☐ Repetitive Strain Injury	☐ Asthma
☐ Amputation	☐ Dislocation	☐ Internal Joint Derangement	☐ Spinal Cord Injury	☐ Cancer
☐ Bite	☐ **Fall from Height**	☐ Joint Effusion	☐ Sprain/Strain	☐ Fumes - Inhalation
☐ Burn	☐ Foreign Body	☐ Laceration	☐ **Surgical Intervention**	☐ Hand-arm Vibration
☐ Contusion/Hematoma/Swelling	☐ **Fracture**	☐ **Neurological Dysfunction**	☐ Tendonitis/Tenosynovitis	☐ Hearing Loss
☐ Crush Injury	☐ Hernia	☐ Psychological	☐▼ Range of Motion	☐ Infectious Disease
	☐ Infection	☐ Puncture (non-needlestick)		☐ Needle Stick
☐ Other				☐ Poisoning/Toxic Effects
				☐ Skin Condition

3. Are you aware of any pre-existing or other conditions/factors that may impact recovery?   ☐ yes ☐ no

If yes, describe _____

4. Diagnosis

D. Treatment Plan

1. What is the treatment plan (type of treatment, duration) including prescribed medications?

2. To be completed by physicians only.

Work Injury/Illness Medications	Dose	Frequency	Duration	Work Injury/Illness Medications	Dose	Frequency	Duration
1.				3.			
2.				4.			

3. Investigations & Referrals:

☐ None ☐ Labs ☐ Xrays ☐ CT Scan ☐ MRI ☐ EMG ☐ Ultrasound ☐ Other _____

☐ FP/GP	☐ Occupational Health Centre	☐ Physiotherapist	Would the patient benefit from the following referrals?
☐ Specialist/Specialty _____	☐ Occupational Therapist	☐ Psychologist	☐ Specialty Clinic
☐ Chiropractor	☐ Other_____		☐ Regional Evaluation Centre (REC)

Name of Referral or Facility (if known)	Telephone	Appointment Date dd mm yyyy

E. Billing Section

Health Professional Designation
☐ Chiropractor ☐ Physician ☐ Physiotherapist ☐ Registered Nurse (Extended Class)

Service Code **8M**   WSIB Provider ID

HST Registration No.	HST Amount Billed (if applicable) $	Service Code **ONHST**	Your Invoice No.	Service Date dd mm yyyy

Health Professional Name (please print)   Address

Telephone   Fax

APPENDIX 9.11

WSIB Functional Abilities Form for Planning Early and Safe Return to Work (Form FAF)

wsib ONTARIO

Mail to:
200 Front Street West
Toronto ON M5V 3J1

or Fax to:
416 344-4684
OR 1-888-313-7373

Please PRINT in black ink

FAF

Functional Abilities Form
for Planning Early
and Safe Return to Work

Claim No.

A. Section A to be completed by the employer and/or worker.

Worker's Last Name

First Name

Telephone

Address (no., street, apt.)

City/Town

Province

Postal Code

Employer's Name

Full Address (No., Street, Apt.)

City/Town   Prov.   Postal Code

Date of Birth
(dd/mm/yyyy)

Date of Accident/
Awareness of Illness
(dd/mm/yyyy)

Employer
Telephone

Employer
Fax No.

1. Type of job at time of accident (where available, please attach description of job activities)

Area(s) of injury(ies)/illness(es)

2. Have the worker and the employer discussed Return To Work

☐ yes   ☐ no

If no, will be discussed on   dd   mm   yyyy

3. Employer contact name

Position

B. Worker's Signature

By signing below, I am authorizing any health professional who treats me to provide me, my employer and the Workplace Safety and Insurance Board (WSIB) with information about my functional abilities on the WSIB's "Functional Abilities for Planning Early and Safe Return to Work" form.

Signature

Please print form & sign before returning to the WSIB

Date   dd   mm   yyyy

C. Health Professional's Billing Information
For billing purposes fax or mail pages 2 and 3 to the WSIB.

Health Professional's Designation

☐ Chiropractor   ☐ Physician   ☐ Physiotherapist   ☐ Registered Nurse (Extended Class)   ☐ Other ___

PROVIDER BILLING INFORMATION IN THE BOLDED AREA OF SECTION C SHOULD NOT BE PROVIDED TO THE WORKER OR EMPLOYER.

Are you registered with the WSIB?
☐ yes   Please enter the **WSIB Provider ID.** in the box provided
☐ no   Please call **1 - 800-569-7919** to register ►

WSIB Provider ID.

Your Invoice Number

Service Code   **FAF**

▼ Complete these fields if **HST** is applicable to this form ▼

HST Registration Number | Service Code | HST Amount Billed

ONHST $.

Health Professional's Name (please print)

Address (No. Street, Apt.)

City/Town   Province   Postal Code   Fax

I hereby declare that the information being submitted in Sections C, D, E and F of this form is true and complete. It is an offense to knowingly make a false or misleading statement or representation to the WSIB.

Health Professional's Signature

Please print form & sign before returning to the WSIB

Telephone

Date   dd   mm   yyyy

2647A2 (07/06)

wsib
ONTARIO

Mail to:
200 Front Street West
Toronto ON M5V 3J1

or Fax to:
416 344-4684
OR 1-888-313-7373

Please PRINT in black ink

FAF

Functional Abilities Form
for Planning Early
and Safe Return to Work

Worker's Last Name	First Name	Claim No.

D. The following information should be completed by the Health Professional to identify the patient's overall abilities and restrictions.

1. Date of Assessment   dd   mm   yyyy

2. Please check one:

▶ ☐ Patient is capable of returning to work with **no restrictions.**

☐ Patient is capable of returning to work **with restrictions.** Complete sections **E and F.**

☐ Patient is physically unable to return to work at this time. Complete section **F.**

E. Abilities and/or Restrictions

1. Please indicate **Abilities** that apply. Include additional details in section 3

Walking:
☐ Full abilities
☐ Up to 100 metres
☐ 100 - 200 metres
☐ Other (please specify)

Standing:
☐ Full abilities
☐ Up to 15 minutes
☐ 15 - 30 minutes
☐ Other (please specify)

Sitting:
☐ Full abilities
☐ Up to 30 minutes
☐ 30 minutes - 1 hour
☐ Other (please specify)

Lifting from floor to waist:
☐ Full abilities
☐ Up to 5 kilograms
☐ 5 - 10 kilograms
☐ Other (please specify)

Lifting from waist to shoulder:
☐ Full abilities
☐ Up to 5 kilograms
☐ 5 - 10 kilograms
☐ Other (please specify)

Stair climbing:
☐ Full abilities
☐ Up to 5 steps
☐ 5 - 10 steps
☐ Other (please specify)

Ladder climbing:
☐ Full abilities
☐ 1 - 3 steps
☐ 4 - 6 steps
☐ Other (please specify)

Travel to work:
Ability to use public transit
☐ yes
☐ no

Ability to drive a car
☐ yes
☐ no

2. Please indicate **Restrictions** that apply. Include additional details in section 3

☐ Bending/twisting repetitive movement of (please specify)

☐ Work at or above shoulder activity:

☐ Chemical exposure to:

☐ Environmental exposure to: (e.g. heat, cold, noise or scents)

☐ Limited use of hand(s):
Left   Right
☐ Gripping ☐
☐ Pinching ☐
☐ Other (please specify) ☐

☐ Limited pushing/pulling with:
☐ Left arm
☐ Right arm
☐ Other (please specify)

☐ Operating motorized equipment: (e.g. forklift)

☐ Potential side effects from medications (please specify) Do not include names of medications.

☐ Exposure to vibration:
☐ Whole body
☐ Hand/Arm

3. Additional Comments on **Abilities and/or Restrictions.**

4. From the date of this assessment, the above will apply for approximately:
☐ 1 - 2 days ☐ 3 - 7 days ☐ 8 - 14 days ☐ 14 + days

5. Have you discussed return to work with your patient?
☐ yes ☐ no

6. Recommendations for work hours and start date:
☐ Regular full-time hours ☐ Modified hours ☐ Graduated hours
Start Date   dd   mm   yyyy

F. Date of Next Appointment

Recommended date of next appointment to review **Abilities and/or Restrictions.**
▶   dd   mm   yyyy

I have provided this completed Functional Abilities Form to: ☐ **Worker**   and/or   ☐ **Employer**

2647A3 (07/06)

SOURCE: Used with permission of WSIB.

Transcribing Orders as a Unit Clerk

10

LEARNING OUTCOMES

After completing this chapter, you should be able to:

- understand the role of the unit clerk
- set up hospital charts for new patients
- record information and data in medical hospital charts
- understand the coloured flag system as it applies to hospital charts
- understand the transcription process
- identify and use medical symbols and abbreviations correctly
- transcribe physicians' orders correctly
- recognize and interpret different laboratory/test requisitions
- understand the medication administration record (MAR)

*To know what has to be done, then do it,
comprises the whole philosophy of practical life.*

—William Osler

Introduction

As a medical office administrator (MA), one of the career paths you may choose is that of a unit clerk. A unit clerk is responsible for reception and clerical tasks—in particular, maintaining patients' charts—on a particular unit within a hospital, thus allowing nurses more time for patient care. In the final chapter of this text, we will look at the MA's role as unit clerk, and at the contents and organization of patients' charts in a hospital. Our focus will be on the clinical data that the unit clerk is responsible for throughout a patient's hospital stay, and how this information is organized and transcribed to complete the patient's chart.

Role of the Unit Clerk

The unit clerk is a vital part of the hospital health care team. A unit clerk performs many duties similar to those of an MA employed in a doctor's office—for example, answering phones, relaying messages, and handling patient inquiries. In addition to these responsibilities, unit clerks do the following:

- Assemble new patient charts.
- Check current and closed patient charts for completeness.
- Transcribe physicians' orders for treatments and medications.
- Complete orders for consultation requests and laboratory diagnostic requisitions.
- File laboratory and test results in patient charts.
- Prepare documentation associated with patient admissions, transfers, discharges, and deaths.
- Coordinate the transportation of patients, specimens, and other materials necessary for patient care.
- Order supplies, such as paper, chart forms, requisition slips, latex gloves, and equipment for the unit.
- In general, act as a central information point for staff, families, and visitors.

> **DID YOU KNOW?**
>
> The unit/ward clerk position was created at the end of the Second World War to provide support for nursing staff by taking on many of the administrative duties associated with patient care, freeing nurses to focus on patients.

A unit clerk's shift is often extremely busy, particularly during the day, and the clerk must excel in multitasking to succeed in this demanding role. Unit clerks work on shift rotation so that there is a unit clerk on each hospital ward 24 hours a day, seven days a week. You must be prepared to work any of the shift rotations. A shift may be 8 or 12 hours. Eight-hour shifts are scheduled from 7:00 a.m. to 3:00 p.m., 3:00 p.m. to 11:00 p.m., and 11:00

p.m. to 7:00 a.m., while 12-hour shifts are scheduled from 7:00 a.m. to 7:00 p.m. (day shift) and 7:00 p.m. to 7:00 a.m. (evening shift).

The unit clerk works at the nurses' station, a centrally located area on each ward where activities are coordinated, information and records are kept, and patients' charts are located. A **ward** is the area on a hospital floor where patients' rooms are located. Each ward is usually specific to a division of medicine, for example, maternity ward, endoscopy ward, general surgery, or osteopathy.

The unit clerk must be familiar with the different types of laboratory, surgical, and diagnostic departments within a hospital setting. He or she will be responsible for transcribing diagnostic, procedure, and laboratory orders onto the correct requisitions. In order to complete this task, the unit clerk must be familiar with the many requisitions and their corresponding departments. In this chapter, we will discuss some of the requisitions a unit clerk will be required to process during the course of a shift, and provide examples.

After an order has been transcribed to the correct requisition, the unit clerk must send a copy of the requisition to the pertinent health care professional or lab technician, and ensure that the testing is scheduled. The unit clerk must also develop his or her own method for confirming that the test was completed and that the results have been received and placed in the patient's chart. At the completion of an order, there also may be specimens or films that the unit clerk might need to send out to an external lab or specialist.

Upon arrival for a shift, a unit clerk will begin by organizing the workspace, filing any reports that have not yet been placed in patients' charts, checking patients' charts for newly written orders, and checking for any new admissions, discharges, or transfers. The unit clerk should also take note of the nursing assignment sheet because knowing which nurses are assigned to which patients will be useful when communicating with staff. For example, if during the physician's rounds the doctor makes a change to a patient's medication, the unit clerk should let the nurse responsible for that patient know that a new medication order has been transcribed to the patient's chart and needs to be initialled.

At the beginning of every shift, the incoming unit clerk will meet with the unit clerk whose shift is ending regarding admissions, discharges, orders waiting to be transcribed, and any special instructions that will need to be processed during the shift. The transcription of orders is not the same as the medical transcription carried out by an MA in a medical office. An MA in a medical office will transcribe a physician's audio recordings detailing patient encounters, whereas a unit clerk transcribes specific medication and treatment instructions directly into patients' charts for prompt action. You will learn more about this difference as the chapter progresses.

After the physicians have completed their rounds, they will leave written orders containing information related to patient care for the unit clerk to transcribe to each patient's chart, for example, information regarding activity, medications, tests, and so on. The orders are typically written by the **most responsible physician (MRP)**, and may be blank, pre-printed, or an **order set**. Pre-printed and set orders save physicians valuable time, but still allow the physician to edit the orders as needed. For an example of a blank, completed physician order (i.e., not pre-printed or part of an order set), see Appendix 10.1.

While the tasks that unit clerks complete are similar for every shift (see the bulleted list on the previous page), the pace on the evening and night shifts is often slower, allowing the unit clerk more time to complete tasks that the day-shift unit clerk may have set aside to complete later—for example, filling in lab requisitions, organizing consultations, booking in-hospital tests, and arranging for porters for the following day. Always remember that any new orders must be processed first. The evening or night-shift clerk will not be able to complete referrals or fill medication requests, as the pharmacy and administrative offices will not be open during these hours.

PRACTICE TIP

If more than one doctor is caring for a hospitalized patient, there is a chance that duplicate or conflicting orders may be written for that patient. Always clarify any discrepancies. Generally, the MRP's orders will be followed. However, before disregarding or overriding any orders, check with the MRP or the physician who wrote them.

ACTIVITIES

1. Test your knowledge: Using the sample physician orders in Appendix 10.1, identify whether the item will be placed on a requisition, the Kardex, or the MAR. Check your answers using Appendix 10.2.

2. Transcribe the following physician orders for Mr. Black onto the correct form. The forms can be found in the Appendixes. Some orders will be placed on more than one form.

PT. DEMOGRAPHICS:

CR#032951

Mr. Robert Black

123 Duncan Street

Kingston, ON K7L 3T5

Male

DOB: September 22, 1947

Religion: RC

HC#3238494232

Family Physician: Dr. V. Patel

ALLERGY: PENICILLIN

Physician's Orders

- CBC
- Electrolytes
- Urine for C&S
- Valium 5 mg po hs
- Lasix 20 mg od
- MS Contin 100 mg IM stat
- Captopril 12.5 mg bid
- Eltroxin 0.1 mg od
- Demerol 50–75 mg IM q4h prn
- Gravol 50 mg q4h prn
- BRP
- IV TKVO Saline
- NPO x 48 hrs
- Ab u/s
- Consult infection control
- Signature and date: Vinayek Patel, October 15, 2014 @1000

ADDITIONAL INFORMATION:

Next of Kin: Black, Elvira

Pt. admitted to Davies 4, Rm. 421

3. Transcribe the physician's orders for Mr. N. Lucky and indicate where each item will be placed.

PT. DEMOGRAPHICS:

CR#000281

Lucky, N.T.

35 Barts Place

Kingston, ON K7T 3V4

Male

DOB: October 8, 1968

Religion: C of E

HC#2194302857

Family Physician: Ku T., Dr.

ALLERGY: SULFA

Physician's Orders

- Vitals q2h
- IV 1000 NS c̄ 20 KCl alt c̄ 1000 S5W c̄ 20 KCl @ 125mL/h
- NPO
- Flagyl 500 mg IV q6h
- Netilmycin 50 mg IV q6h
- Foley catheter
- Isotope scan of kidneys
- CBC & lytes in a.m.
- Signature/Date: Ku, T., October 31, 2014 @09:00

Physician's Orders

- OR in a.m.
- Laparotomy, drainage of abd. abscess and insertion of subclavian line
- T&C x 2 u p.c.
- Vitals q4h, notify MD if T > 39°C
- Maintain IV @ 125 mL/h
- Urine output q/h, notify if > 30 mL/h
- Signature/Date: Ku, T., November 1, 2014 @ 20:00

Physician's Orders

- CBC, lytes in a.m.
- IV to 150 mL/h
- Bolus c̄ 250 mL NS now
- Signature/Date: K. Hawkins, clinical clerk, November 1, 2014 @ 22:00

ADDITIONAL INFORMATION:

Mr. N.T. Lucky has been admitted from the ER with recurrent and abscesses 2° to gunshot wounds.

Next of Kin: Lucky, R.U.—Sister

Admitting Date: October 31, 2014

History: Abdominal pain in L inguinal region, over past 12 h, gradually worsening; nausea, emesis, and anorexia

Admitted to Connell 5 Rm# 521 by Dr. T. Ku.

4. Consider the following discharge orders for Mr. Lucky:

DISCHARGE ORDERS

November 8, 2014:

- D/C home
- TWB R leg and maintain in extension until ortho F/U
- F/U with family doc on POD#14 for staple removal
- F/U with consultant in 6/52 in # clinic
- Scripts attached to chart

J. McClerk

J. McClerk^{cc} 58973

---

    a. What will you need to do before you transcribe the order?

    b. Complete a discharge plan based on the order, spelling out each instruction.

APPENDIX 10.1

Sample Completed Physician's Order Form

HOPE GENERAL HOSPITAL	ADDRESSOGRAPH
Ottawa, ON	
PHYSICIAN'S ORDERS	
WEIGHT KG	DRUG SENSITIVITIES

Please use ballpoint pen. Press firmly to make copy. Thank you.

DATE	TIME	ORDER AND SIGNATURE	TRANSCRIPTION
		CBC	
		Electrolytes	
		Urine for C&S	
		Valium 5 mg po hs	
		Lasix 20 mg od	
		Demerol 100 mg IM stat	
		Enalapril 5 mg bid	
		Eltroxin 0.1 mg od	
		Demerol 50–75 mg IM q4h prn	
		Gravol 50 mg q4h prn	
		BRP	
		NAS x 48 hrs	
		Consult cardiology control	
		Dr. V. Patel, July 6, 2014	
		@10:00 h	

APPENDIX 10.2

Filled-in Physician's Orders Showing Transcription of Items

HOPE GENERAL HOSPITAL		ADDRESSOGRAPH	
Ottawa, ON			
PHYSICIAN'S ORDERS			
WEIGHT	KG	DRUG SENSITIVITIES	

Please use ballpoint pen. Press firmly to make copy. Thank you.

DATE	TIME	ORDER AND SIGNATURE	TRANSCRIPTION
		CBC	First 3 items will be transcribed to a laboratory requisition
		Electrolytes	
		Urine for C&S	
		Valium 5 mg po hs	MAR; routine
		Lasix 20 mg od	MAR; routine
		Demerol 100 mg IM stat	MAR; STAT
		Enalapril 5 mg bid	MAR; routine
		Eltroxin 0.1 mg od	MAR; routine
		Demerol 50–75 mg IM q4h prn	MAR; PRN
		Gravol 50 mg q4h prn	MAR; PRN
		BRP	These 3 items will be transcribed to the Kardex; consultation for cardiology will also require a consultation requisition
		NAS x 48 hrs	
		Consult cardiology control	
		Dr. V. Patel, July 6, 2014	Physician's signature, date, and time
		@10:00 h	

APPENDIX 10.3

Sample Blank Patient Profile/Kardex

PATIENT PROFILE

DEMOGRAPHIC

PREFERRED NAME:

CONTACT PERSON: RELATIONSHIP:

TELEPHONE: RELIGION:

DX: ADMISSION DATE:

PROCEDURE:

HX:

ALLERGIES: ☐ NONE KNOWN ☐ YES

DISCHARGE PLANNING: CODE STATUS:

COLLABORATIVE PLANNING

DATE	DISCIPLINE

DIAGNOSTIC TESTS

DATE	DONE	DATE	DONE

LINES

DATE IN					

PATIENT PROFILE

PATIENT CARE ACTIVITIES	DATE	INTERVENTIONS

COGNITIVE / PERCEPTUAL   INDEPENDENT ☐
- ☐ NEURO V/S _____
- ☐ HEARING AID _____
- ☐ GLASSES / CONTACTS
- COMMUNICATION: ☐ ENGLISH   ☐ OTHER _____
- ☐ SKIN CARE
- ☐ MOOD, AFFECT, BEHAVIOUR _____

RESPIRATION / CIRCULATION   INDEPENDENT ☐
- ☐ TPR _____   ☐ BP _____
- ☐ DB&C _____   ☐ O₂ _____
- ☐ SUCTION _____
- ☐ TRACH _____

NUTRITION   INDEPENDENT ☐
- ☐ FEEDS SELF WITH HELP   ☐ WT _____
- ☐ TOTAL FEED BY STAFF   ☐ DENTURES
- ☐ INTAKE   ☐ CALORIE COUNT
- ☐ DIET _____
- ☐ TPN _____   ☐ SNACK _____
- ☐ NG TUBE _____   ☐ SUCTION _____

ELIMINATION   INDEPENDENT ☐
- ☐ TOILETS WITH HELP   ☐ BED PAN
- ☐ TOILETS WITH CONSTANT SUPERVISION   ☐ COMMODE
- ☐ OUTPUT   ☐ WASHROOM
- INCONTINENT CARE: ☐ PARTIAL   ☐ TOTAL
- ☐ CBI _____
- ☐ CATHETER TYPE _____
- ☐ OSTOMY

MEDICATION ADMINISTRATION RECORD

ROUTINE/SCHEDULED MEDICATIONS

REMARKS:

ROUTINE MEDICATIONS	DOSE	FREQUENCY		Time	Initial	Time	Initial	Time	Initial	Time	Initial	Time	Initial	Time	Initial
ORIGINAL ORDER DATE:															
		1 2 3 4 5 6													
		7 8 9 10 11 12													
		13 14 15 16 17 18													
REORDER DATE:		19 20 21 22 23 24													
	ROUTE:														
ORIGINAL ORDER DATE:															
		1 2 3 4 5 6													
		7 8 9 10 11 12													
		13 14 15 16 17 18													
REORDER DATE:		19 20 21 22 23 24													
	ROUTE:														
ORIGINAL ORDER DATE:															
		1 2 3 4 5 6													
		7 8 9 10 11 12													
		13 14 15 16 17 18													
REORDER DATE:		19 20 21 22 23 24													
	ROUTE:														
ORIGINAL ORDER DATE:															
		1 2 3 4 5 6													
		7 8 9 10 11 12													
		13 14 15 16 17 18													
REORDER DATE:		19 20 21 22 23 24													
	ROUTE:														
ORIGINAL ORDER DATE:															
		1 2 3 4 5 6													
		7 8 9 10 11 12													
		13 14 15 16 17 18													
REORDER DATE:		19 20 21 22 23 24													
	ROUTE:														
ORIGINAL ORDER DATE:															
		1 2 3 4 5 6													
		7 8 9 10 11 12													
		13 14 15 16 17 18													
REORDER DATE:		19 20 21 22 23 24													
	ROUTE:														
ORIGINAL ORDER DATE:															
		1 2 3 4 5 6													
		7 8 9 10 11 12													
		13 14 15 16 17 18													
REORDER DATE:		19 20 21 22 23 24													
	ROUTE:														

MEDICATION ADMINISTRATION RECORD

PRN/UNSCHEDULED MEDICATIONS

REMARKS:

PRN MEDICATIONS	DOSE	FREQUENCY	Time	Initial	Time	Initial	Time	Initial	Time	Initial	Time	Initial	Time	Initial
ORIGINAL ORDER DATE:														
		INDICATIONS:												
REORDER DATE:														
	ROUTE:													
ORIGINAL ORDER DATE:														
		INDICATIONS:												
REORDER DATE:														
	ROUTE:													
ORIGINAL ORDER DATE:														
		INDICATIONS:												
REORDER DATE:														
	ROUTE:													
ORIGINAL ORDER DATE:														
		INDICATIONS:												
REORDER DATE:														
	ROUTE:													
ORIGINAL ORDER DATE:														
		INDICATIONS:												
REORDER DATE:														
	ROUTE:													
ORIGINAL ORDER DATE:														
		INDICATIONS:												
REORDER DATE:														
	ROUTE:													
ORIGINAL ORDER DATE:														
		INDICATIONS:												
REORDER DATE:														
	ROUTE:													

MEDICATION ADMINISTRATION RECORD

CONTINUOUS PARENTERAL MEDICATIONS

ORDER DATE	CONTINUOUS PARENTERAL MEDICATIONS e.g., potassium, heparin, insulin, etc.	ROUTE	TRANSFER	CHECK	START			DISCONTINUED		
					Date	Time	Initial	Date	Time	Initial

APPENDIX 10.5

Sample Blank Laboratory Requisition

HOPE GENERAL HOSPITAL
77 Gladview Avenue, Ottawa, ON K2S 3G8
613-813-1234 [telephone]   info@hgh.emp.ca
613-813-1235 [fax]   www.hgh.emp.ca

LABORATORY REQUISITION

[If in a setting that has an addressograph, imprint patient information here.]

Please bring your requisition and OHIP card to your appointment. Arrive at least 15 minutes prior to scheduled appointment.

Requisitioning Practitioner		Address

Facility No.	CPSO No.	Clinician/Practitioner's Contact Number for Urgent Results

Name (as it appears on Health Card)

Sex ☐ M ☐ F	Date of Birth (yyyy mm dd)	Service Date

Address		Postal Code
Home Phone	Work Phone	Cell Phone

Check One   ☐ OHIP/Insured   ☐ Third Party/Uninsured   ☐ WSIB

Health Card Number (OHIP)	Version Code (if applicable)

Card Expiry Date (if applicable)

BIOCHEMISTRY	HEMATOLOGY	Viral Hepatitis (check one only)
☐ Glucose ☐ Random ☐ Fasting	☐ CBC	☐ Acute Hepatitis
☐ HbA1C	☐ Prothrombin Time (INR)	☐ Chronic Hepatitis
☐ TSH	**IMMUNOLOGY**	☐ Immune Status/Previous Exposure
☐ Creatinine (eGFR)	☐ Pregnancy test (Urine)	Specify ☐ Hepatitis A
☐ Uric Acid	☐ Mononucleosis Screen	☐ Hepatitis B
☐ Sodium	☐ Rubella	☐ Hepatitis C
☐ Potassium	☐ Prenatal: ABO, RhD, Antibody Screen (titre and ident. If positive)	Or order individual hepatitis tests in the "Other Tests" section below
☐ Chloride	☐ Repeat Prenatal Antibodies	
☐ CK		
☐ ALT	**Microbiology ID & Sensitivities (if warranted)**	**Prostate Specific Antigen (PSA)**
☐ Alk. Phosphate	☐ Cervical	☐ Total PSA ☐ Free PSA
☐ Bilirubin	☐ Vaginal	☐ Insured Meets OHIP eligibility criteria
☐ Albumin	☐ Vaginal/Rectal – Group B Strep	☐ Uninsured - Screening Patient responsible for paying
☐ Lipid Assessment Includes Cholesterol, HDL-C, Triglycerides, calculated LDL-C & Chol/HDL-C ratio; individual lipid tests may be ordered in the "Other Tests" sections of this form.	☐ Chlamydia (specify source)	**Vitamin D (25-Hydroxy)**
	Source	☐ Insured Meets OHIP eligibility criteria: osteopenia; osteoporosis; rickets; renal disease; malabsorption syndromes; medications affecting vitamin D metabolism
	☐ GC (specify source)	
	Source	
	☐ Sputum	
☐ Vitamin B12	☐ Throat	
☐ Ferritin	☐ Wound (specify source)	☐ Uninsured - Screening Patient responsible for paying
☐ Albumin/Creatinine Ratio, Urine	Source	
☐ Urinalysis (Chemical)	☐ Urine	**Other Tests**
☐ Ferritin	☐ Stool Culture	
☐ Neonatal Bilirubin: Child's age: days hours Clinician/practitioner's phone #: Patient's 24-hour phone #:	☐ Stool Ova & Parasites	
	☐ Other Swabs/Pus (specify source)	
	Source	
	Specimen Collection	
	Time	Date	
	Fecal Occult Blood Test (FOBT) (check one)	
Therapeutic Drug Monitoring	FOBT (non CCC)	
Name of Drug 1	Colon Cancer Check (FOBT) CCC	
Name of Drug 2	*Laboratory Use Only*	
Time Collected Drug 1 (hr)		
Time of Last Dose 1 (hr)		
Time of Next Dose 1 (hr)		
I hereby certify the tests ordered are not for a registered patient of Hope General on an inpatient or outpatient basis		
Signature		

APPENDIX 10.6

Sample Laboratory Requisition Results

```
Client:                Patient Name:              Accession #:  WN7342694
              726      Birthdate:                 Sex: F
              12         Phone #:  (613)
                        Health #:
                                        Date of service:  26-November-14
                                               Printed:  01-December-14
Requesting physician:  Dr. Fred Anyone          Reference #:
                                          Report status:  FINAL
```

TEST NAME	RESULT	ABNORMAL	REFERENCE RANGE	UNITS	TEST LOG #
*HEMOGLOBIN	124	✓	120 – 160	g/L	XO
*HEMATOCRIT	0.38		0.35 – 0.45		
*WHITE BLOOD CELL COUNT	5.2		4.0 – 11.0	x E9/L	
*RED BLOOD CELL COUNT	4.08	✓	4.00 – 5.10	x E12/L	
*MCV	92.4		80 – 95	fL	
*MCH	30.4		27.5 – 33.0	pg	
*MCHC	328		320 – 360	g/L	
*RDW	13.6		11.5 – 14.5		
*PLATELET COUNT	272		150 – 400	x E9/L	
*ABSOLUTE: NEUTS	3.5		2.0 – 7.5	x E9/L	
* (A) LYMPH	1.3		1.0 – 3.5	x E9/L	
* (A) MONO	0.4		0.0 – 0.8	x E9/L	
* (A) EOS	0.0		0.0 – 0.5	x E9/L	
* (A) BASO	0.0		0.0 – 0.2	x E9/L	
*RBC	NO ABNORMALITIES DETECTED BY INSTRUMENT				
*WBC	NO ABNORMALITIES DETECTED BY INSTRUMENT				
*PLATELETS	NO ABNORMALITIES DETECTED BY INSTRUMENT				
*GLUCOSE-RANDOM	5.0		3.6 – 6.9	MMOL/L	
*THYROTROPIN (SENSITIVE TSH)	1.33		0.35 – 5.00	MIU/L	10
NA	142		135 – 145	MMOL/L	
K	4.6		3.5 – 5.0	MMOL/L	
CL	105		98 – 107	MMOL/L	
URIC ACID	6.0		2.5 – 7.5	MG/DL	

```
                           FINAL REPORT
      PND = Pending     * = Not previously reported     ~ = Edited result
```

APPENDIX 10.7

Sample Blank Discharge Plan

DISCHARGE PLAN

HOPE GENERAL HOSPITAL
77 Gladview Avenue, Ottawa, ON   K2S 3G8
613-813-1234 [telephone]   info@hgh.emp.ca
613-813-1235 [fax]   www.hgh.emp.ca

PHARMACIST'S COPY

DIET:

ACTIVITY:

CLINIC APPT: LOCATION:

DR.   DATE: TIME:

SEE YOUR FAMILY DOCTOR:

HOME CARE REFERRAL: ☐YES ☐NO

PUBLIC HEALTH NURSE REFERRAL: ☐YES ☐NO

PATIENT'S PHONE:

DIAGNOSIS AND REASON FOR REFERRAL TO PHN:

INSTRUCTIONS TO PATIENT:

OTHER MEDICATIONS (NOT ON PRESCRIPTION):

COMPLETED BY: STATUS:

DISCHARGE DATE:

DATE:

PRESCRIPTION:

DOCTOR'S SIGNATURE:

DOCTOR'S NAME (PRINT):

PATIENT INSTRUCTION SUMMARY

TOPIC	REMARKS	DATE	SIGNATURE

APPLICATION FOR CONTINUING CARE (to be completed by social worker)

NAME	LEVEL	DATE SENT	DATE ASSESSED	DATE APPROVED	DATE OF TRANSFER
1.					
2.					
3.					
4.					

ECIS APPLICATION #: _____ SENT: _____ RECEIVED: _____ SOCIAL WORKER: _____

ACTUAL DISCHARGE DATE: _____ TO: _____ HOW: _____

DISCHARGE PLAN

APPENDIX 10.8

Filled-in Discharge Plan

DISCHARGE PLAN

DIET: *As tolerated*

ACTIVITY: *Bed rest with bathroom privileges first week, then up as normal*

CLINIC APPT: *In 3 weeks*   LOCATION:

DR.   DATE: TIME:

SEE YOUR FAMILY DOCTOR:

HOME CARE REFERRAL: ☐ YES ☐ NO

PUBLIC HEALTH NURSE REFERRAL: ☐ YES ☐ NO

PATIENT'S PHONE:

DIAGNOSIS AND REASON FOR REFERRAL TO PHN:

INSTRUCTIONS TO PATIENT: *Abdominal pain resolved. Continue with medications as directed. Limit activity first week home, then resume regular activity as tolerated. If symptoms of nausea, vomiting, anorexia, and lower right quadrant pain return go to the ER*

OTHER MEDICATIONS (NOT ON PRESCRIPTION):

COMPLETED BY: *A Gutelius*   STATUS: *RN*

DISCHARGE DATE: *July 9, 2014*

HOPE GENERAL HOSPITAL
77 Gladview Avenue, Ottawa, ON K2S 3G8
613-813-1234 [telephone]   info@hgh.emp.ca
613-813-1235 [fax]   www.hgh.emp.ca

PHARMACIST'S COPY

DATE: *July 9, 2014*

PRESCRIPTION:

Metronidazole 2000 mg, by mouth, once a day for 14 days

DOCTOR'S SIGNATURE: *G. Hanson*

DOCTOR'S NAME (PRINT):   *GARY HANSON*

PATIENT INSTRUCTION SUMMARY

TOPIC	REMARKS	DATE	SIGNATURE

APPLICATION FOR CONTINUING CARE (to be completed by social worker)

NAME	LEVEL	DATE SENT	DATE ASSESSED	DATE APPROVED	DATE OF TRANSFER
1.					
2.					
3.					
4.					

ECIS APPLICATION #: _____ SENT: _____ RECEIVED: _____ SOCIAL WORKER: _____

ACTUAL DISCHARGE DATE: _____ TO: _____ HOW: _____

DISCHARGE PLAN

APPENDIX 10.9

Sample Blank Discharge Sheet

DISCHARGE SHEET

ADMITTED:

YYYY/MM/DD   TIME

DISCHARGED:

YYYY/MM/DD   TIME

NO ABBREVIATIONS TO BE USED

HOPE GENERAL HOSPITAL
77 Gladview Avenue, Ottawa, ON K2S 3G8
613-813-1234 [telephone]   info@hgh.emp.ca
613-813-1235 [fax]   www.hgh.emp.ca

MOST RESPONSIBLE DX: DIAGNOSIS MOST RESPONSIBLE FOR HOSPITAL STAY:

OTHER PRIMARY DIAGNOSIS INFLUENCING LENGTH OF STAY:

COMPLICATIONS ARISING DURING HOSPITALIZATION:

OTHER SECONDARY CONDITIONS (THAT DID NOT INFLUENCE LENGTH OF STAY):

CODE

MEDICAL RECORDS USE ONLY

	TRANSFERS		
	SERV.	DR.	DAYS
SPEECH			
A.L.C.			
CL NUT.			
O.T.			
P.T.			
R.T.			
S.W.			
DIS. PL.			
OTHER			

DATE PERFOMED			PROCEDURES	CODE
YYYY	MM	DD		*MEDICAL RECORDS USE ONLY*

WARNING HISTORY OF UNTOWARD REACTION TO ▶

DISCHARGE MEDICATIONS / FOLLOW UP / OTHER INSTRUCTIONS

DISCHARGE DESTINATION

ARRANGEMENTS FOR FUTURE CARE	SEND COPY OF THE SUMMARY TO	NAME
☐ FAMILY DOCTOR	☐ ▶	
☐ REFERRING DOCTOR	☐ ▶	
☐ ATTENDING DOCTOR	☐ ▶	
☐	☐ ▶	
☐	☐ ▶	

FINAL SUMMARY

DICTATED BY:

DATE:

S I G N E D

_____ MD
RESIDENT

_____ MD
ATTENDING DOCTOR

APPENDIX 10.10

ISMP's List of Error-Prone Abbreviations, Symbols, and Dose Designations

The abbreviations, symbols, and dose designations found in this table have been reported to the Institute for Safe Medication Practices (ISMP) through the ISMP National Medication Errors Reporting Program (ISMP MERP) as being frequently misinterpreted and involved in harmful medication errors. They should NEVER be used when communicating medical information. This includes internal communications, telephone/verbal prescriptions, computer-generated labels, labels for drug storage bins, medication administration records, as well as pharmacy and prescriber computer order entry screens.

Abbreviations	Intended Meaning	Misinterpretation	Correction
μg	Microgram	Mistaken as "mg"	Use "mcg"
AD, AS, AU	Right ear, left ear, each ear	Mistaken as OD, OS, OU (right eye, left eye, each eye)	Use "right ear," "left ear," or "each ear"
OD, OS, OU	Right eye, left eye, each eye	Mistaken as AD, AS, AU (right ear, left ear, each ear)	Use "right eye," "left eye," or "each eye"
BT	Bedtime	Mistaken as BID (twice daily)	Use "bedtime"
cc	Cubic centimetres	Mistaken as "u" (units)	Use "mL"
D/C	Discharge or discontinue	Premature discontinuation of medications if D/C (intended to mean "discharge") has been misinterpreted as "discontinued" when followed by a list of discharge medications	Use "discharge" and "discontinue"
IJ	Injection	Mistaken as IV or "intrajugular"	Use "injection"
IN	Intranasal	Mistaken as IM or IV	Use "intranasal" or "NAS"
HS hs	Half-strength At bedtime, hours of sleep	Mistaken as "bedtime" Mistaken as "half-strength"	Use "half-strength" or "bedtime"
IU*	International unit	Mistaken as IV (intravenous) or 10 (ten)	Use "units"
o.d. or OD	Once daily	Mistaken as "right eye" (OD; oculus dexter), leading to oral liquid medications being administered in the eye	Use "daily"
OJ	Orange juice	Mistaken as OD or OS (right or left eye); drugs meant to be diluted in orange juice may be given in the eye	Use "orange juice"
Per os	By mouth, orally	The "os" can be mistaken as "left eye" (OS; oculus sinister)	Use "PO," "by mouth," or "orally"
q.d. or QD*	Every day	Mistaken as q.i.d., especially if the period after the "q" or the tail of the "q" is misunderstood as an "i"	Use "daily"
qhs	Nightly at bedtime	Mistaken as qhr (every hour)	Use "nightly"
qn	Nightly or at bedtime	Mistaken as qh (every hour)	Use "nightly" or "at bedtime"
q.o.d. or QOD*	Every other day	Mistaken as q.d. (daily) or q.i.d. (four times daily) if the "o" is poorly written	Use "every other day"
q1d	Daily	Mistaken as q.i.d. (four times daily)	Use "daily"
q6PM, etc.	Every evening at 6 p.m.	Mistaken as "every 6 hours"	Use "daily at 6 p.m." or "6 p.m. daily"
SC, SQ, sub q	Subcutaneous	SC mistaken as SL (sublingual); SQ mistaken as "5 every"; the "q" in "sub q" has been mistaken as "every" (e.g., a heparin dose ordered "sub q 2 hours before surgery" misunderstood as every 2 hours before surgery)	Use "subcut" or "subcutaneously"

Abbreviations	Intended Meaning	Misinterpretation	Correction
ss	Sliding scale (insulin) or 1/2 (apothecary)	Mistaken as "55"	Spell out "sliding scale"; use "one-half" or "1/2"
SSRI SSI	Sliding scale regular insulin Sliding scale insulin	Mistaken as selective serotonin reuptake inhibitor Mistaken as "strong solution of iodine" (Lugol's)	Spell out "sliding scale (insulin)"
i/d	One daily	Mistaken as "tid"	Use "1 daily"
TIW or tiw	3 times a week	Mistaken as "3 times a day" or "twice in a week"	Use "3 times weekly"
U or u*	Unit	Mistaken as the number 0 or 4, causing a 10-fold overdose or greater (e.g., 4U seen as "40" or 4u seen as "44"); mistaken as "cc" so dose given in volume instead of units (e.g., 4u seen as 4cc)	Use "unit"
UD	As directed (ut dictum)	Mistaken as unit dose (e.g., "diltiazem 125 mg IV infusion UD" misinterpreted to mean giving the entire infusion as a unit [bolus] dose)	Use "as directed"

Dose Designations and Other Information	Intended Meaning	Misinterpretation	Correction
Trailing zero after decimal point (e.g., 1.0 mg)*	1 mg	Mistaken as 10 mg if the decimal point is not seen	Do not use trailing zeros for doses expressed in whole numbers
"Naked" decimal point (e.g., .5 mg)*	0.5 mg	Mistaken as 5 mg if the decimal point is not seen	Use zero before a decimal point when the dose is less than a whole unit
Abbreviations such as mg. or mL. (with a period following the abbreviation)	mg mL	The period is unnecessary and could be mistaken as the number 1 if written poorly	Use mg, mL, etc. without a terminal period
Drug name and dose run together (especially problematic for drug names that end in "l," such as Inderal40 mg; Tegretol300 mg)	Inderal 40 mg Tegretol 300 mg	Mistaken as Inderal 140 mg Mistaken as Tegretol 1300 mg	Place adequate space between the drug name, dose, and unit of measure
Numerical dose and unit of measure run together (e.g., 10mg, 100mL)	10 mg 100 mL	The "m" is sometimes mistaken as a zero or two zeros, risking a 10- to 100-fold overdose	Place adequate space between the dose and unit of measure
Large doses without properly placed commas (e.g., 100000 units; 1000000 units)	100,000 units 1,000,000 units	100000 has been mistaken as 10,000 or 1,000,000; 1000000 has been mistaken as 100,000	Use commas for dosing units at or above 1,000, or use words, such as "100 thousand" or "1 million" to improve readability

To avoid confusion, do not abbreviate drug names when communicating medical information. Examples of drug name abbreviations involved in medication errors include:

Drug Name Abbreviations	Intended Meaning	Misinterpretation	Correction
APAP	acetaminophen	Not recognized as acetaminophen	Use complete drug name
ARA A	vidarabine	Mistaken as cytarabine (ARA C)	Use complete drug name
AZT	zidovudine (Retrovir)	Mistaken as azathioprine or aztreonam	Use complete drug name
CPZ	Compazine (prochlorperazine)	Mistaken as chlorpromazine	Use complete drug name
DPT	Demerol-Phenergan-Thorazine	Mistaken as diphtheria-pertussis-tetanus (vaccine)	Use complete drug name
DTO	Diluted tincture of opium, or deodorized tincture of opium (Paregoric)	Mistaken as tincture of opium	Use complete drug name

Drug Name Abbreviations	Intended Meaning	Misinterpretation	Correction
HCl	hydrochloric acid or hydrochloride	Mistaken as potassium chloride (the "H" is misinterpreted as "K")	Use complete drug name unless expressed as a salt of a drug
HCT	hydrocortisone	Mistaken as hydrochlorothiazide	Use complete drug name
HCTZ	hydrochlorothiazide	Mistaken as hydrocortisone (seen as HCT250 mg)	Use complete drug name
MgSO4*	magnesium sulphate	Mistaken as morphine sulphate	Use complete drug name
MS, MSO4	morphine sulphate	Mistaken as magnesium sulphate	Use complete drug name
MTX	methotrexate	Mistaken as mitoxantrone	Use complete drug name
PCA	procainamide	Mistaken as patient-controlled analgesia	Use complete drug name
PTU	propylthiouracil	Mistaken as mercaptopurine	Use complete drug name
T3	Tylenol with codeine No. 3	Mistaken as liothyronine	Use complete drug name
TAC	triamcinolone	Mistaken as tetracaine, adrenaline, cocaine	Use complete drug name
TNK	TNKase	Mistaken as "TPA"	Use complete drug name
ZnSO4	zinc sulphate	Mistaken as morphine sulphate	Use complete drug name

Stemmed Drug Names	Intended Meaning	Misinterpretation	Correction
"Nitro" drip	nitroglycerin infusion	Mistaken as sodium nitroprusside infusion	Use complete drug name
"Norflox"	norfloxacin	Mistaken as Norflex	Use complete drug name
"IV Vanc"	intravenous vancomycin	Mistaken as Invanz	Use complete drug name

Symbols	Intended Meaning	Misinterpretation	Correction
℥	Dram	Symbol for dram mistaken as "3"	Use the metric system
♍	Minim	Symbol for minim mistaken as "mL"	Use the metric system
x3d	For three days	Mistaken as "3 doses"	Use "for three days"
> and <	Greater than and less than	Mistaken as the opposite of intended; mistakenly use incorrect symbol; "<10" mistaken as "40"	
/ (slash mark)	Separates two doses or indicates "per"	Mistaken as number 1 (e.g., "25 units/10 units" misread as "25 units and 110 units"	
@	At	Mistaken as "2"	
&	And	Mistaken as "2"	
+	"Plus" or "and"	Mistaken as "4"	
°	Hour	Mistaken as a zero (e.g., "q2°" seen as "q 20")	
Φ or ⊘	Zero or null sign	Mistaken as numbers 4, 6, 8, and 9	

* These abbreviations are included on The Joint Commission's "minimum list" of dangerous abbreviations, acronyms, and symbols that must be included on an organization's "Do Not Use" list, effective January 1, 2004. Visit www.jointcommission.org for more information about this Joint Commission requirement.

SOURCE: Reproduced from the Institute for Safe Medication Practices. http://www.ismp.org/tools/errorproneabbreviations.pdf. Used with permission.

APPENDIX 10.11

Sample Blank Parenteral Nutrition Order

HOPE GENERAL HOSPITAL
77 Gladview Avenue, Ottawa, ON K2S 3G8
613-813-1234 [telephone]   info@hgh.emp.ca
613-813-1235 [fax]   www.hgh.emp.ca

PHYSICIAN'S ORDERS

WEIGHT (KG)   DRUG SENSITIVITIES

PLEASE USE BALLPOINT PEN AND PRESS FIRMLY.
NOTE: ORDERS MUST BE RECEIVED IN PHARMACY BY 1300H, OTHERWISE SOLUTIONS WILL BE SUPPLIED FOR THE FOLLOWING DAY.

ORDER AND SIGNATURE: PARENTERAL NUTRITION ORDER FORM (ADULT ICU)	Transcription & RN Notes
☐ New Order (complete Section A and Section B) ☐ Continue Enteral Nutrition (EN) _____ (solution) at 10 mL/h ☐ Order Modification (complete only Section B) ☐ Initiate Adult ICU Glycemic Control Protocol (physician to complete an Adult ICU Glycemic Control Protocol order form)	
☐ **SECTION A: New Parenteral Nutrition (PN) Orders**	
1. Consult Clinical Dietician (required for all initial orders).	
2. CBC, platelets, INR, PTT, blood glucose, electrolytes, calcium, phosphate, magnesium, urea, creatinine, triglycerides, serum albumin, AST, alkaline phosphatase, total bilirubin.	
3. Twice weekly weights (every Monday and Thursday).	
4. Monitor intake/output q12 h.	
5. Initiate amino acid and dextrose infusion IV at _____ mL/h for 6 hours, then increase by 25 mL/h every 6 hours if blood glucose is less than 9 mmol/L until target PN rate reached (as ordered in Section B).	
6. **DAILY** electrolytes and blood glucose until patient has received PN for 5 days at target PN rate.	
7. **TWICE WEEKLY** (every Monday and Thursday) calcium, magnesium, phosphate, urea, creatinine, prealbumin, electrolytes and blood glucose.	
8. **WEEKLY** (every Monday) CBC, AST, alkaline phosphatase, total bilirubin, triglycerides, serum albumin, 24 hour urinary urea and creatinine clearance	
☐ **SECTION B: New or Modified Parenteral Nutrition (PN) orders (refer to the Calculation of Adult Daily Energy Requirements on reverse)**	
1. Base solution: (select one) ☐ Amino acids 5% and dextrose 25% (central) at target PN rate of _____ mL/h **OR** ☐ Amino acids 5% and dextrose 16.6% (central) at target PN rate of _____ mL/h **OR** ☐ Amino acids 4.25% and dextrose 10% (central/peripheral) at target PN rate of _____ mL/h **OR** ☐ Other (consult pharmacy): _____ at target PN rate of _____ mL/h	
2. Electrolytes: ☐ Standard: Calcium 2.25 mmol/L **OR** ☐ Non-Standard: Calcium _____ mmol/L Magnesium 2.5 mmol/L Magnesium _____ mmol/L Sodium 35 mmol/L Sodium _____ mmol/L Potassium 40 mmol/L Potassium _____ mmol/L Phosphate 15 mmol/L Phosphate _____ mmol/L	
3. Multivitamins IV – one dose daily. Trace elements IV – one dose daily.	
4. ☐ Vitamin K _____ mg IV/IM once weekly on Fridays.	
5. If PN is longer ☐ Fat emulsion 20% 250 mL IV **OR** ☐ Fat emulsion 20% IV than 1 week: at 20 mL/h once a week. at _____ mL/h.	
6. ☐ Glutamine 15 grams PO/NG tid.	
7. Other orders:	

PHYSICIAN SIGNATURE   PRINTED NAME   DATE & TIME

Original – Chart   Copy – Pharmacy   Physician's Orders

APPENDIX 10.12

Special Order Sample: Respiratory Care

**RESPIRATORY THERAPY
ORDER FORM**

(Patient Label)
Room

DIRECTIONS FOR COMPLETING FORM

1. All orders for Respiratory Therapy <u>MUST</u> be written on this Respiratory Therapy Order Form, except orders for Mechanical Ventilation, which must be written on the Mechanical Ventilation Form.
2. Select therapy below that corresponds with appropriate indication.
3. For consultation: Inability to take deep breaths or stridor — contact Respiratory Therapy Department: Ext. 55901 or beeper #91601.

PHYSICIAN ORDER

NOTE: All therapy is discontinued after 7 days. Physician must evaluate respiratory therapy orders before reordering.

BRONCHODILATOR THERAPY   *See reverse side for additional information on HHN/MDI conversion and titration protocol.*

Modality determined by Respiratory Therapist according to Respiratory Therapy Policy #036.1

☐ Albuterol Titration: Respiratory Therapy to titrate dose and frequency according to clinical assessment and Respiratory Therapy Policy #036.1

☐ Albuterol   ☐ Ipratoplum Bromide   ☐ Racemic Epinephrine

☐ Other Medication: _____

Initial Dose and Frequency: _____

OXYGEN/HUMIDITY THERAPY   *See reverse side for additional information.*

Indication:

☐ Hypoxemia or risk for hypoxemia
(Documentation of SaO_2 <93% or PaO_2 <70 mmHg on room air is required within 72 hours.)

☐ Thick, tenacious secretions, unable to clear spontaneously

☐ Patients with tracheostomy or endotracheal tube (off ventilator) } Aerosol: ☐ Cool ☐ Heated

☐ Other _____

Delivery system _____ L/M _____ or FIO2   ☐ Keep O_2 Saturation: _____ %

MONITORING / MEASUREMENTS / DIAGNOSTICS

☐ Diagnostic sputum induce with Hypertonic Saline (10%), patient is not spontaneously productive

☐ Peak Expiratory Flow Rate   ☐ Vital Capacity

☐ Wearing Parameters   ☐ Other (specify): _____

Frequency: _____

DISCONTINUE: _____

PHYSICIAN SIGNATURE	DATE	TIME	PAGER
NURSE (ORDER SIGN-OFF)	DATE	TIME	
RESPIRATORY THERAPIST (ORDER SIGN-OFF)	DATE	TIME	

APPENDIX 10.13

Filled-in Patient Profile/Kardex

PATIENT PROFILE

NPO 13/10 @ 0700 h   SULFA

DEMOGRAPHIC

PREFERRED NAME: Not Too Lucky

CONTACT PERSON: R.U. Lucky   RELATIONSHIP: Sister

TELEPHONE: 613-547-9056   RELIGION: RC

DX: Abd abscess 2° to gunshot wounds   ADMISSION DATE: Oct. 13, 2014

PROCEDURE: Laparotomy – drainage of abscess

Insertion of subclavian line

HX: Abd pain in (L)inguinal region over past 24 h

gradually worsening; nausea, emesis, and anorexia

ALLERGIES: ☐ NONE KNOWN ☑ YES   SULFA

DISCHARGE PLANNING:

CR#00281
NT Lucky
35 Barts Place
Kingston ON K1T 3Y4
DOB: August 10, 1968/M
HC 274302857

COLLABORATIVE PLANNING

DATE	DISCIPLINE
15/10	Laparotomy to drain abd abscess
	Insertion of subclavian line

CODE STATUS:

DIAGNOSTIC TESTS

DATE	Labs	DONE
13/10	CBC } in AM	
13/10	Lytes	
14/10	T:C x 20	

DATE	Procedures/Tests	DONE
13/10	Foley catheter	
13/10	Isotope scan of kidneys	
15/10	Laparotomy	
15/10	Subclavian line	

LINES

DATE IN	
Oct 13	1000 mL NS c̄ 20 kcl alt c
Oct 13	1000 mL D5N c̄ 20 kcl 125 mL/h
Oct 14	? Bolus c̄ 500 mL NS @ 2000
	Maintain 125 mL/L
Oct 15	Maintain IV @ 125/h

PATIENT PROFILE

PATIENT CARE ACTIVITIES	DATE	INTERVENTIONS
COGNITIVE / PERCEPTUAL INDEPENDENT ☐		
☐ NEURO V/S		
☐ HEARING AID		
☐ GLASSES / CONTACTS		
COMMUNICATION: ☐ ENGLISH ☐ OTHER _____		
☐ SKIN CARE		
☐ MOOD, AFFECT, BEHAVIOUR _____	Oct 13	q. 2 h 0900 h
RESPIRATION / CIRCULATION INDEPENDENT ☐	Oct 14	q. 4 h 2000 h
☑ TPR 2 q. h q. 4 h ☐ BP _____		notify MD if T > 37°C
☐ DB&C ☐ O₂ _____		
☐ SUCTION		
☐ TRACH		
NUTRITION INDEPENDENT ☐		
☐ FEEDS SELF WITH HELP ☐ WT	Oct 13	NPO 0900 h
☐ TOTAL FEED BY STAFF ☐ DENTURES		
☐ INTAKE ☐ CALORIE COUNT		
☐ DIET NPO		
☐ TPN ☐ SNACK _____		
☐ NG TUBE ☐ SUCTION _____		
ELIMINATION INDEPENDENT ☐		
☐ TOILETS WITH HELP ☐ BED PAN		
☐ TOILETS WITH CONSTANT SUPERVISION ☐ COMMODE		
☐ OUTPUT ☐ WASHROOM		
INCONTINENT CARE: ☐ PARTIAL ☐ TOTAL		
☐ CBI	Oct 13	0900 h
☑ CATHETER TYPE Foley	Oct 14	2000 q. h notify MD if urine output > 30 mL / h
☐ OSTOMY		

PATIENT PROFILE

PATIENT CARE ACTIVITIES	DATE	INTERVENTIONS

SKIN HYGIENE   INDEPENDENT ☐

☐ BATHES WITH ASSISTANCE   ☐ EYE CARE _____
☐ BATHED BY STAFF   ☐ MOUTH CARE _____
☐ BED BATH   ☐ PERI CARE _____
☐ TUB / SHOWER   ☐ SKIN CARE _____
☐ SHAMPOO   ☐ WOUND _____

MOBILITY   AAT ☐   INDEPENDENT ☐

TOTAL / PARTIAL ASSISTANCE, NUMBER OF STAFF, FREQUENCY

☐ BED REST _____
☐ ASSIST TO CHAIR _____
☐ ASSIST TO WALK _____
☐ TOTAL ASSIST TO TURN / 008 _____
☐ AIDS / LIFTS _____
☐ ROM EXERCISES _____

SAFETY   INDEPENDENT ☐

BED RAILS ☐ UPPER ☐ LOWER   ☐ LT ☐ RT
           ☐ CONTINUOUS   ☐ NIGHT ONLY

RESTRAINTS: _____

OBSERVATION: _____
_____
_____

☐ SLEEP / REST
☐ SOCIAL / ECONOMIC
☐ REPRODUCTION / SEXUALITY
☐ SPIRITUAL
☐ INFECTION CONTROL
☐ PAIN MANAGEMENT

ROOM#: *Cornell 521*   NAME: *N.T. Lucky*   AGE: *45*   PHYSICIAN: *Dr. Ky. T.*

PAGE 3 OF 3

APPENDIX 10.14

Filled-in Medication Administration Record (MAR)

HOPE GENERAL HOSPITAL
77 Gladview Avenue, Ottawa, ON   K2S 3G8
613-813-1234 [telephone]   613-813-1235 [fax]
info@hgh.emp.ca   www.hgh.emp.ca

NPO   SULFA   CR#00281
NT Lucky
35 Barts Place
Kingston   ON   K1T 3Y4
HC 2194302857
DOB: August 10, 1968 / M

MEDICATION ADMINISTRATION RECORD (LONG FORM)

ONE DOSE ONLY, PREOPERATIVE, AND STAT MEDICATIONS

_____1___ of _____1___ booklets

| ORDER DATE | ONE DOSE ONLY, PRE-OP, AND STAT MEDICATIONS | ROUTE | TRANSFER | CHECK | GIVEN | | ADMIN BY |
					DATE	TIME	
Oct 12	Bolus 500 mL & NS	IV	AU				
@ 2000h	Maintain IV @ 125 mL / h						

Recopied ☐   Date: _____

NPO   SULFA   NT Lucky
35 Barts Place
Kingston ON K1T 3Y4
HC 2194302857
DOB: August 10, 1968 / M

MEDICATION ADMINISTRATION RECORD

ROUTINE/SCHEDULED MEDICATIONS

REMARKS:

ROUTINE MEDICATIONS	DOSE	FREQUENCY		Oct 13		Oct 14		Oct 15		Oct 16		Oct 17		Oct 18	
				Time	Initial	Time	Initial	Time	Initial	Time	Initial	Time	Initial	Time	Initial
ORIGINAL ORDER DATE: Oct 13 Flagyl REORDER DATE:	500mg	q. 6h 1 2 3 4 5 ⑥ 7 8 9 10 11 ⑫ 13 14 15 16 17 ⑱ 19 20 21 22 23 ㉔													
		ROUTE: IV AU													
ORIGINAL ORDER DATE: Oct 13 Netilmycin REORDER DATE:	50mg	q. 6h 1 2 3 4 5 ⑥ 7 8 9 10 11 ⑫ 13 14 15 16 17 ⑱ 19 20 21 22 23 ㉔													
		ROUTE: IV AU													
ORIGINAL ORDER DATE: REORDER DATE:		1 2 3 4 5 6 7 8 9 10 11 12 13 14 15 16 17 18 19 20 21 22 23 24													
		ROUTE:													
ORIGINAL ORDER DATE: REORDER DATE:		1 2 3 4 5 6 7 8 9 10 11 12 13 14 15 16 17 18 19 20 21 22 23 24													
		ROUTE:													
ORIGINAL ORDER DATE: REORDER DATE:		1 2 3 4 5 6 7 8 9 10 11 12 13 14 15 16 17 18 19 20 21 22 23 24													
		ROUTE:													
ORIGINAL ORDER DATE: REORDER DATE:		1 2 3 4 5 6 7 8 9 10 11 12 13 14 15 16 17 18 19 20 21 22 23 24													
		ROUTE:													
ORIGINAL ORDER DATE: REORDER DATE:		1 2 3 4 5 6 7 8 9 10 11 12 13 14 15 16 17 18 19 20 21 22 23 24													
		ROUTE:													

APPENDIX 10.15

Filled-in Parenteral Medication Order on Medication Administration Record (MAR)

NPO   SULFA   *NT Lucky*
35 Barts Place, Kingston ON K1T 3Y4

MEDICATION ADMINISTRATION RECORD   *HC 2194302857*

CONTINUOUS PARENTERAL MEDICATIONS   *DOB: August 10, 1968 / M*

ORDER DATE	CONTINUOUS PARENTERAL MEDICATIONS e.g., potassium, heparin, insulin, etc.	ROUTE	TRANSFER	CHECK	START Date	START Time	START Initial	DISCONTINUED Date	DISCONTINUED Time	DISCONTINUED Initial
Oct 13	*PCA–IU AU*	*IU*	*AU*							

Glossary

A

accessibility *Canada Health Act* requirement that provinces must provide reasonable access to insured health services on uniform terms and conditions, without financial or other barriers

addressograph address labelling machine

alphanumeric filing filing system composed of sequential letters and numbers

anaphylaxis allergic reaction that causes dramatic vascular and bronchial changes leading to respiratory distress (trouble breathing)

annotating method of summarizing or highlighting the key information in a document

attending physician physician who is primarily responsible for the hospital care of a patient

B

blended capitation model payment scheme in which physicians receive a base payment per patient. However, each physician is also able to receive incentives and special payments for the provision of specific primary health care services. The base payment amount is calculated by taking the physician's enrollment and multiplying it by the capitation rate.

blended salary model payment scheme in which physicians are salaried employees of an organization or community-sponsored family health team, and their salary is based on the number of rostered patients to each individual physician. Bonuses and special payments may be achieved through the provision of specific primary health care services—e.g., ensuring that every patient on the roster has an up-to-date immunization record.

block fee flat fee charged for a predetermined set of uninsured services, such as telephone prescription renewal; also called an "annual fee"

brand name proprietary or trade name of a drug, copyrighted by the manufacturer

C

Canada Health Act federal legislation for publicly funded health care insurance

capacity ability (a) to understand the information that is relevant to deciding whether to consent to the collection, use, or disclosure of personal information, and (b) to appreciate the reasonably foreseeable consequences of giving, not giving, withholding, or withdrawing such consent

capitation method of payment for health services by which a group is prepaid a fixed, per capita amount for each patient served, without considering the actual amount of the service provided to each patient by the GP

charge-out system system to keep track of charts when they have been removed for purposes other than for use while the patient is in the medical office or hospital

chemical name unique designation describing a drug's atomic or molecular structure; e.g., the chemical name for Lasix is 4-chloro-2-(furan-2-ylmethylamino)-5-sulfamoylbenzoic acid

chemistry panel group of tests routinely ordered to determine a person's general health status based on a blood sample

cluster scheduling method of organizing appointments whereby similar procedures are performed at the same time or day of the week—e.g., all physicals are booked for Thursday afternoons; also called "affinity scheduling."

coding physical act of marking correspondence for filing; e.g., the MA may underline or write a code word on the document to demonstrate where it should be filed

combination scheduling method of organizing appointments that combines open scheduling with cluster scheduling. Some appointments are combined by similarity (e.g., physical and pre-operative exams), with the rest being booked at any time; also called "blended scheduling."

community care access centres (CCACs) in Ontario, local agencies that provide information about care options, enabling ill or aged people to live independently at home

complement-based base remuneration compensation based on the number of physicians within a family practice group and their commitment to offering regular and reasonable extended office hours. This compensation model offers a base remuneration plus funding to meet overhead costs accrued in managing the services within the community.

complete blood count (CBC) test that determines the number of white blood cells, red blood cells, and platelets in a patient's bloodstream

comprehensiveness *Canada Health Act* requirement that plans must cover all medically necessary services provided by doctors and hospitals

critical thinking skills ability to consider all aspects of a situation or conflict when deciding what action to take

cross-referencing method of managing charts and documentation that allows the MA to connect one chart to another—e.g., in the case of patients who change their name, or when it is difficult to distinguish a first name from a surname

cystic pertaining to a cyst—i.e., a raised, solid mass filled with liquid

D

de-identify with regard to personal health information, removing any details that could be used to identify an individual—e.g., name, date of birth, OHIP number

diagnostic code alphanumeric list of codes used to group and identify diseases, disorders, symptoms, and medical signs; used for a physician's billing purposes

diagnostic test test that identifies a disease based on its signs and symptoms

double booking scheduling two patients in the same time slot for the same provider

downtime time during the day when routine work is completed, allowing the MA to address backlogs, assist a co-worker, or otherwise help the office to function

E

edema condition characterized by swelling due to excess fluid collecting in body cavities or tissues

efficacy capacity for producing a desired result or effect

electronic health record (EHR) computerized medical record for a specific patient that can be shared with more than one health care organization

electronic medical record (EMR) computerized medical record for a specific patient that can be shared within a single health care organization

enrollment act of joining a family health care practice as a patient. Patients agree to visit their family doctor or group first when in need of medical treatment, allow the provincial ministry of health to share personal health information with their physician or family practice group, and not to change physicians or family practice groups more than twice per year

ergonomics study of the relationship between humans and their work environments

ethics moral principles that govern individual or group behaviour

express consent consent that is clearly and unmistakably stated; it may be given in writing, orally, or non-verbally— e.g., by a clear gesture such as a nod

extra-billing the billing of an insured health service by a medical practitioner in an amount greater than the amount paid or to be paid for that service by the provincial or territorial health insurance plan

F

fee codes alphanumeric listing of physician service codes that describe the length of patients' visits and the fee that the physician will receive

fee-for-service remuneration method of payment in which the patient or insurance company pays the physician for professional services according to a specific schedule of fees

filing process of organizing health records on a shelf, in a filing cabinet, or in an electronic database

fixed office hours system of patient appointments in which the doctor is available at regular times (e.g., 9:00 a.m. to 4:00 p.m.) and sees patients at previously booked appointment times; also called "open scheduling" or "stream scheduling"

fluoroscope instrument with a fluorescent screen, used for viewing X-ray images without taking and developing X-ray photographs

Freedom of Information and Protection of Privacy Act **(FIPPA)** Ontario legislation requiring the government to protect the privacy of personal information contained in its records, including the collection, retention, use, disclosure, and disposal of personal information; and to provide public access to government data, including general records and records that contain personal information

G

generic name non-proprietary name by which a drug is known; e.g., the generic name for Lasix is "furosemide"

geographic filing method of record keeping in which documents are filed alphabetically within categories arranged according to geographic locations

H

hCG (human chorionic gonadotropin) pregnancy hormone hormone that becomes elevated after conception

health claim, health care payment (HCP) claim filed for services rendered by a physician or private medical lab to a patient who has Ontario health insurance

hiatal hernia protrusion of an organ, typically the stomach, through the esophageal opening in the diaphragm

home care supportive care provided in patients' homes; also called "community care"

I

imaging visual representation of an object, such as a body part, for the purpose of medical diagnosis

implied consent consent that is not expressly granted, but rather inferred from a person's actions and the facts and circumstances of a particular situation—e.g., rolling up one's sleeve to receive an injection

indexing method of organizing a filing system, whether alphabetically (by subject or geographically), numerically, or alphanumerically

international normalized ratio (INR) blood testing done in combination with other tests to determine the ability of a patient's blood to clot

intrathecal pertaining to the space surrounding the brain and spinal cord that contains cerebrospinal fluid (CSF)

ionizing radiation radiation that can harm human health when absorbed by the body—e.g., X-rays

L

law rule of conduct or action that is prescribed or formally recognized as binding and is enforced by a controlling authority

local health integration networks (LHINs) in Ontario, 14 regional health care agencies that plan, integrate, and fund local health care

locum physician who temporarily assumes another physician's clinical duties—e.g., while the latter is on holiday or extended leave

long-term care municipal or charitable nursing homes for the aged, chronically ill, or disabled; some offer respite care or short-stay care

M

medical records any record of a patient's medical information, whether in printed form, on film, by electronic means or otherwise, including correspondence, memorandum, book, plan, map, drawing, diagram, pictorial or graphic work, photograph, film, microfilm, sound recording, videotape, machine-readable record, or any other documentary material, regardless of physical form or characteristics, and any copy thereof (based on FIPPA, s. 2(1)); also called a "chart"

medicare in Canada, government-funded health care insurance covering doctors' fees and other medically necessary services

midstream sterile urine sample, obtained when the patient voids a small amount, wipes the area with an antiseptic wipe, and then voids into the receptacle

modified wave scheduling method of scheduling appointments in which two patients are seen at regular intervals within a given hour—e.g., every 30 minutes

most responsible diagnosis (MRD) the condition most responsible for hospitalization

most responsible physician (MRP) the physician who has final responsibility and is accountable for the medical care of a patient

musculoskeletal disorders (MSDs) injuries or pain in the body's joints, ligaments, muscles, nerves, tendons, or structures that support the limbs, neck, and back

O

online booking automated tool that allows patients to book appointments online

open office hours scheduling system of patient appointments in which the doctor is available at regular times (e.g., 9:00 a.m. to 4:00 p.m.) and sees patients in the order in which they arrive

open office scheduling system of appointments in which patients are seen whenever they want to be seen; requires holding open a strategic number of time slots for same-day appointments

opt in a physician's choice to bill under the provincial medical insurance plan

opt out a physician's choice not to bill under the provincial plan but to bill the patient directly. The physician must not bill the patient more than the amount set out by the provincial ministry of health for the service.

oral glucose tolerance test (OGTT) measure of the body's ability to use glucose, a sugar that is the body's main source of energy. An OGTT can be used to diagnose prediabetes and diabetes. The test is most commonly done during pregnancy to check for gestational diabetes.

order set grouped medical orders that help regulate diagnosis and treatment of specific illnesses or diseases. Such checklists help maintain a standard of patient care across the hospital and physicians—e.g., a physician order set for care of stroke patients.

P

parenteral medications drugs intended for administration as an injection or infusion—e.g., intravenously (into a vein), subcutaneously (under the skin), or intramuscularly (into muscle); infusions typically are given by the intravenous route

partial thromboplastin time (PTT) measure of the time required to form a clot in a blood sample

personal health information (PHI) identifiable information in oral or written form relating to an individual's health and health care history—e.g., OHIP number; diagnostic, treatment, and care information; information related to payment for health care services

***Personal Health Information Protection Act* (PHIPA)** Ontario legislation that requires health care personnel to safeguard patients' personal health information against theft, loss, and unauthorized disclosure or use; to access only the information they need to do their job; and to keep medical records accurate and up to date

personal health record (PHR) electronic medical record used by the patient to keep track of past and future medical appointments, lists of medications and treatments, correspondence with health care providers, and an immunization schedule; it may take the form of emails, electronic calendars for tracking appointments, and chat rooms for sharing medical information

phlebotomist specialist in obtaining blood samples through venipuncture for purposes of testing, experimentation, or diagnosis

physician's appointment preferences doctor's preferred means of scheduling patients—e.g., physicals only in the afternoon and quick checks between 8:00 a.m. and 11:00 a.m.

portability *Canada Health Act* requirement that a province must continue to cover its residents when they travel elsewhere in Canada

potency with regard to a drug, the amount (dose) needed to produce the desired effect, such as pain relief

practical skills technical or administrative skills—e.g., word processing, use of spreadsheets and billing software, filing

pregnancy test strip medical test that detects the hCG hormone in urine to determine whether a female is pregnant

prescription medicinal preparation made or dispensed according to directions written to a pharmacist by a physician or other authorized health care professional

primary care care that a patient receives at first contact with the health care system, usually involving coordination of care and continuity over time; often provided by a physician, but also by nurses

problem-oriented medical record (POMR) method of arranging patient charts, in reverse chronological order, to reflect the action to be taken on each complaint and the patient's progress in response to treatment

procedure and policy manual written guide describing office routines and practices

prophylaxis agent used to protect or prevent disease or pregnancy

prothrombin time (PT) test to determine the time required for blood to clot

public administration *Canada Health Act* requirement that health care insurance plans must be operated on a non-profit basis by a public authority

public health units (PHUs) agencies established by municipalities to promote health and disease prevention; they deliver programs in schools and other organizations covering such topics as healthy lifestyles, sexual health, vaccinations, addictions, growth and development, parenting education, and screening services

R

radiology study of radiographs; in a health care facility, the department responsible for maintaining radiological equipment and records, and analyzing diagnostic films

reciprocal medical billing (RMB) claim claim billed for services rendered by a physician or private medical lab to a patient insured under another Canadian provincial health plan outside Ontario, excluding Quebec

referral the directing of a patient to a medical specialist by a primary care physician

Remittance Advice explanation of physician remuneration that comes from OHIP

repetitive stress injuries (RSIs) injuries affecting tendons, tendon sheaths, muscles, nerves, and joints; they cause persistent or recurring pains most commonly in the neck, shoulders, forearms, hands, wrists, elbows, and lower limbs

reverse chronological order method of organizing documentation by placing items with the most recent date or number on top or in front

rostering patient registration with a family physician or group; allows the family practice, the province, and the federal government to track patient demographics

S

salaried model payment scheme in which a physician's salary is based on the patient population. Salaried physicians are employees of community health centres providing care to a specific patient population.

secondary care treatment by a specialist to whom a patent has been referred by a primary care provider

Snellen chart eye chart commonly used to test vision; letters on the chart are arranged from smallest to largest

SOAP abbreviation for *Subjective* complaints, *Objective* findings, *Assessment* of findings, and *Plan* for treatment; a method of structuring a chart note

soft skills attributes that enable a person to interact effectively and harmoniously with others—e.g., good communication and listening skills, self-motivation, empathy, cultural sensitivity, ability to think critically

source-oriented medical records (SOMRs) method of organizing patient charts into sections according to subject matter or source of origin; e.g., all lab reports together, all progress reports together

subject filing alphabetic arrangement of records filed by topic or grouped under a common theme

T

telemedicine electronically enabled medical practice, including diagnosis and consultation via telephone or web camera, such as monitoring of vital signs, diabetes, asthma, and home dialysis; computer-assisted surgery; and public health awareness and education

terminal digit filing method of information storage that groups all files ending in the same two digits into a single section; most commonly used in large filing systems, especially in hospitals, insurance companies, government personnel offices, and financial institutions

tertiary care medical care that involves advanced and complex procedures and treatments, usually over an extended period of time, performed by specialists in state-of-the-art facilities (e.g., hospitals, rehabilitation clinics)

tickler system reminder system of prompts for performing time-sensitive tasks, such as bill payments

U

universality *Canada Health Act* requirement that all residents of a province must be entitled to the benefits of its health care plan

user charge any charge for an insured health service, other than extra-billing, that is permitted by a provincial or territorial health insurance plan and is not payable by the plan

V

visual acuity sharpness of vision

W

ward floor area in a hospital where patients' rooms are located; each ward is usually specific to a branch of medicine—e.g., maternity, endoscopy, general surgery, osteopathy

wave scheduling method of grouping patient appointments at the top of each hour, on the assumption that not everyone will be on time

Workplace Safety and Insurance Board (WSIB) claim for services rendered to patients with Ontario health insurance coverage who have been injured on the job; formerly WCB (Workers' Compensation Board)

Index